Toll-Like Receptors in Vector-Borne Diseases

Authored By

Jayalakshmi Krishnan
Department of Life Sciences,
Central University of Tamil Nadu,
Thiruarvur,
India

Toll-Like Receptors in Vector-Borne Diseases

Author: Jayalakshmi Krishnan

ISBN (Online): 978-981-5124-54-5

ISBN (Print): 978-981-5124-55-2

ISBN (Paperback): 978-981-5124-56-9

First published in 2023.

BENTHAM SCIENCE PUBLISHERS LTD.

End User License Agreement (for non-institutional, personal use)

This is an agreement between you and Bentham Science Publishers Ltd. Please read this License Agreement carefully before using the ebook/echapter/ejournal (**"Work"**). Your use of the Work constitutes your agreement to the terms and conditions set forth in this License Agreement. If you do not agree to these terms and conditions then you should not use the Work.

Bentham Science Publishers agrees to grant you a non-exclusive, non-transferable limited license to use the Work subject to and in accordance with the following terms and conditions. This License Agreement is for non-library, personal use only. For a library / institutional / multi user license in respect of the Work, please contact: permission@benthamscience.net.

Usage Rules:

1. All rights reserved: The Work is the subject of copyright and Bentham Science Publishers either owns the Work (and the copyright in it) or is licensed to distribute the Work. You shall not copy, reproduce, modify, remove, delete, augment, add to, publish, transmit, sell, resell, create derivative works from, or in any way exploit the Work or make the Work available for others to do any of the same, in any form or by any means, in whole or in part, in each case without the prior written permission of Bentham Science Publishers, unless stated otherwise in this License Agreement.
2. You may download a copy of the Work on one occasion to one personal computer (including tablet, laptop, desktop, or other such devices). You may make one back-up copy of the Work to avoid losing it.
3. The unauthorised use or distribution of copyrighted or other proprietary content is illegal and could subject you to liability for substantial money damages. You will be liable for any damage resulting from your misuse of the Work or any violation of this License Agreement, including any infringement by you of copyrights or proprietary rights.

Disclaimer:

Bentham Science Publishers does not guarantee that the information in the Work is error-free, or warrant that it will meet your requirements or that access to the Work will be uninterrupted or error-free. The Work is provided "as is" without warranty of any kind, either express or implied or statutory, including, without limitation, implied warranties of merchantability and fitness for a particular purpose. The entire risk as to the results and performance of the Work is assumed by you. No responsibility is assumed by Bentham Science Publishers, its staff, editors and/or authors for any injury and/or damage to persons or property as a matter of products liability, negligence or otherwise, or from any use or operation of any methods, products instruction, advertisements or ideas contained in the Work.

Limitation of Liability:

In no event will Bentham Science Publishers, its staff, editors and/or authors, be liable for any damages, including, without limitation, special, incidental and/or consequential damages and/or damages for lost data and/or profits arising out of (whether directly or indirectly) the use or inability to use the Work. The entire liability of Bentham Science Publishers shall be limited to the amount actually paid by you for the Work.

General:

1. Any dispute or claim arising out of or in connection with this License Agreement or the Work (including non-contractual disputes or claims) will be governed by and construed in accordance with the laws of Singapore. Each party agrees that the courts of the state of Singapore shall have exclusive jurisdiction to settle any dispute or claim arising out of or in connection with this License Agreement or the Work (including non-contractual disputes or claims).
2. Your rights under this License Agreement will automatically terminate without notice and without the

need for a court order if at any point you breach any terms of this License Agreement. In no event will any delay or failure by Bentham Science Publishers in enforcing your compliance with this License Agreement constitute a waiver of any of its rights.

3. You acknowledge that you have read this License Agreement, and agree to be bound by its terms and conditions. To the extent that any other terms and conditions presented on any website of Bentham Science Publishers conflict with, or are inconsistent with, the terms and conditions set out in this License Agreement, you acknowledge that the terms and conditions set out in this License Agreement shall prevail.

Bentham Science Publishers Pte. Ltd.
80 Robinson Road #02-00
Singapore 068898
Singapore
Email: subscriptions@benthamscience.net

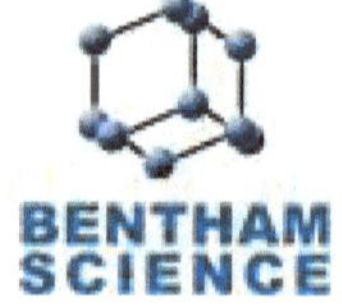

CONTENTS

FOREWORD

This topic is appropriate when we talk about the control of vector-borne diseases as a top priority in the world. Vector-borne diseases are a huge public health problem all over the world. Vectors are organisms that transmit pathogens from infected human to animal or from animal to human, accounting for 17% of Vector-borne diseases (VBDs). Vector-borne diseases such as Malaria, Dengue, Chikungunya, Human African Trypanosomiasis, Leishmaniasis, Japanese encephalitis, Chaga's diseases, Yellow fever, Leishmaniasis, and Onchocerciasis have become major public health concern affecting more than one billion cases and one million deaths globally. There is an urgent need to control these challenges and state of art techniques and science and technology will take it forward. Toll-like receptors are the primary pattern recognition receptors in the human systems and in eliciting innate immune signalling. Cytokines produced through toll-like receptors activation act as a bridge to elicit an adaptive immune response as well. I appreciate this book's title on toll-like receptors in vector-borne diseases as this book can be read by many researchers, industry persons, policymakers, and academicians and can cater to the needs of the research on these vector-borne diseases.

I convey my best wishes to the editor and hope this book will be a great success.

Sangdun Choi
Department of Molecular Science and Technology,
Dean of Graduate School, Ajou University,
Suwon,
Korea

PREFACE

Organisms/animals that transmit diseases are called vectors. They cause serious health problems to the human population such as illness and death. Famous vectors that cause diseases include fleas, ticks, mites, and mosquitos. Mostly, the vectors are invertebrate arthropods and non-living fomites. A disease that can be transmitted from an arthropod or a fomite to a human or animal or plant is called a vector-borne disease (VBDs). Vectors are able to carry and transmit various infectious organisms such as parasites, bacteria and viruses. Vector-borne diseases in a given country affect the socio-economic status and have a huge impact on the Global disease burden.

Ironically, despite decades of research on VBDs, still much remains to be discovered on the complicated relationships between vector, host, and pathogen in their internal environment. The emergence of new diseases such as Zika possess more questions on the complicity of host-pathogen-vector interaction. Any effective vaccine/intervention/ depends on the complete information on the molecules that perform interaction between host-pathoge--vector. Hence, a complete understanding is very much essential. Vector-borne diseases are a threat to the community worldwide. Each year 2.5 billion people in over 100 countries (WHO reports) die of such diseases. Brain inflammation, coma, cerebral leakage, meningitis, neuronal and glial cell degeneration, endothelial dysfunction, blood-brain barrier leakage, and disturbance in Cerebro Spinal Fluid (CSF) circulation have all been noted in various vector-borne diseases such as dengue, Chikungunya, Malaria, West Nile fever, Filariasis and Japanese encephalitis (JE) . I wish our readers can be satisfied with many questions which they feel excited to find the answer for research questions on the etiology of neurological sequale of vector-borne diseases in this book.

Jayalakshmi Krishnan
Department of Life Sciences,
Central University of Tamil Nadu,
Thiruarvur,
India

CHAPTER 1

Introduction to Vector Borne Diseases

Abstract: Vector-borne diseases(VBDs) are reported to represent amount 17% of all infectious diseases. The geographical distribution of vectors depends upon various climatic factors, and social factors. In the recent past, the spread of VBDs across the world is so rapid that it is associated with a change in climatic factors, global warming, travel and trade, unplanned urbanization, deforestation *etc.* Amongst the vector-borne diseases notable is West Nile fever (WNF) caused by West Nile Virus (WNV). WNF belongs to the family of Flaviviridae, which is part of the Japanese encephalitis antigenic group. WNV is transmitted from infected birds to human beings by mosquito bites. WNV is readily reported in Africa, Europe, the Middle East, North America and West Asia. Looking at the history, WNV was first isolated in a woman in the West Nile district of Uganda in 1937. It was identified in birds (crows and columbiformes) in the Nile delta region in 1953. Over the past 50 years, human cases of WNV have been reported in various countries.

Keywords: Chikungunya fever, Dengue, Leishmaniasis, Malaria, Vector-borne diseases (VBDs), West Nile fever (WNF).

INTRODUCTION

Vector-borne diseases(VBD)s are reported to represent amount 17% of all infectious diseases. The geographical distribution of vectors depends upon various climatic factors, and social factors. In the recent past, the spread of VBDs across the world is so rapid that it is associated with change in climatic factors, global warming, travel and trade, unplanned urbanization, deforestation *etc.*

Amongst the vector-borne diseases notable is West Nile fever (WNF) caused by West Nile Virus (WNV). WNF belongs to the family of Flaviviridae which is part of the Japanese encephalitis antigenic group. WNV is transmitted from infected birds to human beings by mosquito bites. WNV is readily reported in Africa, Europe, the Middle East, North America and West Asia. Looking at the history, WNV was first isolated in a woman in the West Nile district of Uganda in 1937. It was identified in birds (crows and columbiformes) in the Nile delta region in 1953. Over the past 50 years, human cases of WNV are reported in various countries.

Jayalakshmi Krishnan

CHIKUNGUNYA

For joint pain caused by chikyngunya medicines such as nacproxen, ibuprofen, and acetaminophen can be tried. Joint pain caused by chikungunya persists for several weeks even after the fever has been cured. As of now there is no vaccine for the treatment of chikyngunya and no antiviral treatment is available. Using insect repellent, sleeping under the mosquito net, breeding places control, wearing full clothes can be used as preventive options for chikungunya.The word Chikungunya is coined from the makondae language which means bends up or contorted "walk with bent over". This disease was reported in 1952 after an outbreak in Makonde Plateau in eastern Tanzania. Initially, this disease was reported seen in Africa and Asia but after 2007, it is also reported to occur from various European countries as well. Currently, more than 60 countries are reporting this fever. The mosquitos which spread Chikungunya fever are day bitters, they spread the disease from one infected person to another normal person when they bite. Symptoms last for 2 to 12 days after the infection begin.The fever is divided into acute and chronic phases,in which the acute phase is known as the febrile phase. Fever is the main symptom in the acute phase and in the chronic phase and is characterised by inflammatory joint pain in some patients up to years it can extend.

Chikungunya fever is a viral disease like WNV that belongs to the genus Alphavirus from the family of *Togaviridae*. Chikungunya fever is transmitted to human beings by the infected mosquito of *Ad aegypti,* and *Ae albopictus*. Chikungunya fever was first described during an outbreak in southern Tanzania in 1952. At present, CHIKV is reported in 50 countries.

LEISHMANIASIS

Leishmaniasis is a protozoan parasitic infection that is transmitted to human beings through the bite of an infected female sandfly. There are three types of Lieshmaniasis, cutaneous, visceral and mucocutaneous. Amongst these, Visceral Lieshmaniasis is progressing rapidly in east Africa with the highest mortality and morbidity. Visceral leishmaniasis if not treated can lead to high rates of mortality and epidemics. Cutaneous leishmaniasis is observed in Afghanistan and Syrian Republic. According to WHO, in 2014, more than 90% of new cases were reported to WHO from six countries: Brazil, Ethiopia, India, Somalia, South Sudan and Sudan. Strikingly, a vast major case of cutaneous Leishmaniasis is reported from Pakistan, Peru, Saudi Arabia and the Syrian Arab Republic, Afghanistan, Algeria, Brazil, Colombia, and the Islamic Republic of Iran. Mucocutaneous leishmaniasis is reported in Bolivia, Brazil and Peru, somewhere around 90%. Surprisingly, the control programs for Kala-azar are successful in

South-East Asia Region (SEARO) countries.

MALARIA

Malaria is caused by one of four species of the *Plasmodium* parasite transmitted by female *Anopheles* spp mosquitoes. Malaria vector control methods have been proven successful in the past which is one of the deadliest vector-borne diseases. Malaria is one of the life-threatening diseases. According to WHO, in 2015 an estimated 212 million cases of malaria occurred worldwide and 429,000 people died, mostly children in the African Region. According to CD, about 1,500 cases of malaria are diagnosed in the United States each year. In India, malaria is a well-known reported public health problem. According to National Vector Bone Diseases Control Programme (NVBDCP), in 2017, among the total of 1,98, 303 cases of malaria, it was reported that *Plasmodium falsiparum* is seen in 1,42,152 cases.

DENGUE

Dengue is the most important arboviral human disease,*Ae. aegypti,* and *Ae. albopictus*, the dengue vectors can be easily influenced by changing humidity, temperature, rainfall, degree of urbanization, and control measures taken by various countries. According to WHO before 1970, dengue was reported in nine countries only, however, now the spread is so rapid that dengue is reported in more than 100 countries, and such a situation is very alarming. In 2016, 1,29,166 cases have been reported in India by the National Vector Borne Disease Control Programme (NVBDCP).

JE was first reported in Uttar Pradesh, the main JE epidemic area in the northern state of India in 1978. The *Cx.vishnui* subgroup, and the *Cx. tritaeniorhynchus, Cx. seudovishnui* and *Anopheles subpictus*, were the main mosquito vectors and secondary vectors in India. In 2016, a total of 1676 cases of JE is reported from India according to NVBDCP. The virus is a single-stranded RNA virus.Pigs and birds are the intermediate hosts of the virus. Human beings are considered dead-end hosts. Upon bite of the infection the virus replicates in the lymph nodes and then viremia develops. After this, the virus enters the central nervous system to effect. The virus has the capacity to alter neurodevelopment also. There is no effective treatment for this viral infection but there can be supportive care and fluids given. Southeast Asian nations and west pacific nations are at higher risk of reporting the cases. Avoiding mosquito bites is the best prevention for this disease.

During rainy seasons the mosquitoes breed a lot and thus increase the chances of disease spread. The JE virus belongs to the *flavivirus* which is related to dengue virus, West nile virus and yellow fever. More than 3 billion people are risk for getting the JE disease. In Japan in 1971 the first case of dengue fever is reported. The incubation period of the virus ranges from four to fourteen days.

The virus was first isolated in 1935, however until now the origin of the virus remains sceptical. Travelling to JE endemic areas can increase the susceptibility of the person to the virus. Immunization can be done to prevent the spread of the virus. The types of vaccines available for JE diseases are: Live recombinant vaccines, live attenuated vaccines, inactivated Vero cell derived vaccines and inactivated mouse brain derived vaccines. The virus spreads only through the bite of the mosquito not from person to person. There is no specific medicine or treatment for this virus but immunization can help and also avoid the mosquito bites by taking preventing measures can help the people in getting the disease. Some animals like birds and pigs can serve as large reservoir of the virus for the spread of the disease through the mosquito bite. The best way to prevent the disease is to wear long sleeved shirts and pants, DEET insect repellents can be used. Early evening walks should be avoided in endemic areas as this time is the greatest activity of the JE mosquitoes. There are five genotypes of Japanese encephalitis virus it has 11 KB single stranded RNA which is of 3800 KD.The infected people first report the non –specific febrile illness followed by lose of consciousness and occurring of convulsions or seizures. Neurological sequel is reported in admitted patients , however around 30% of patients die of the virus induced illness.

CONCLUDING REMARKS

Vector-borne diseases are a public health threat. Increasing cases of these diseases year by year in the world pose a threat to human health and well-being. Mosquitoes such as *Ae.aegypti,* and *Ae.albopictus* spread dengue and CHICKV. The spread of dengue is so rapid that it is reported more than in 100 countries.WNV is reported in Africa, Europe, the middle east, North America and West Asia. Looking at the history, WNV was first isolated in a woman in the west Nile district of Uganda in 1937. All these historical events warn that VBDs are not going to be restricted in one place but going to spread to so many non-endemic areas and hence their control becomes a priority task.

CONSENT FOR PUBLICATION

Not applicable.

CONFLICT OF INTEREST

The author declares no conflict of interest, financial or otherwise.

ACKNOWLEDGEMENT

Declared none.

CHAPTER 2

Pattern Recognition Receptors in Brain: Emphasis on Toll Like Receptors and their Types

Abstract: The immune system is highly complex; it senses foreign invaders, thus protecting the body. The adaptive arm of the immune system confers long-term protection, whereas the innate immune system confers immediate protection. In the case of the immune system, the pattern recognition receptors offer various modes of sensing the pathogen-associated molecular patterns present in pathogens. The receptors that sense invading pathogens are called Pattern recognition receptors [1]. The adaptive immune system is very sophisticated, as it is trained to identify only the "specific antigen", but PPRs are customised to sense a wide array of "common patterns" present in the pathogens. Cerebral pericytes are the cells that are seen as embedded in the basement membrane of capillaries. Matzinger [2] gave a new insight into the recognition of pathogens by PRRs as those that recognise PAMPs and DAMPs (Damage Associated Molecular Patterns). While PAMPs can be presented as exogenous ligands to the receptor, DAMPs are presented as endogenous ligands. Once these PRRs are activated either by PAMPs or DAMPs, they lead to the production of inflammation to clear the infection. However, over-activation during chronic conditions leads to pathological changes.

Keywords: CD 14 cofactor, DAMPs, NF-κB, TLRs.

INTRODUCTION

TLRs can be present in the membrane or in the intracellular system, wherever they are located they can recognise the PAMPs. They are a part of the surveillance system in the cells along with other mechanisms. Viral, bacterial, parasitic and any other pathogenic components can be recognised by TLRs.

There are 13 TLRs that are currently identified and all of them use MyD88 as their adaptor molecule except TLR3 [1, 2]. This activation can produce inflammatory responses through the recruitment of various kinases and adaptor molecules. These include the activation of NF-κB and MAPKs, such as stress-activated protein kinase/JNK and p38. In humans, TLR1-10 are present, whereas in Mice along with the homologues of TLR1-9 there are additional TLRs, *i.e.*, TLR 11 to 13 are present [3 - 5]. Further, ten chicken (avain) functional TLRs are

Jayalakshmi Krishnan

identified [6]. Among these TLRs, TLR3, TLR7-9 and TLR11-13 can be seen in endosomes which are intracellular organelles.

TLR1, 2, 4, 5, 6 and 10 are present in the cell surface. These TLRs differ in their ability to bind and recognise pathogens. Most bacterial ligands can be identified by TLR1, 2, 4, 5, 6, and 10 in which TLR 2 and 4 (CD 14 as a cofactor) can also recognise viral surface proteins [7, 8]. Sometimes, upon pathogenic binding TLRs form either homo or heterodimers [9]. TLR-induced pathways can be bifurcated as two, based on their ability to use myeloid differentiation factor 88 (MyD88). Except for TLR3 all TLRs use the MyD88-dependent pathway, TLRs use the TRIF pathway to entice the inflammatory events.

Brain and Pathogen Associated Molecular Patterns

Brain pericytes have been shown to express a variety of PRRs including TLRs, NOD, and NLRs [10]. Pericytes have been known to control various neurovascular functions such as cerebral blood flow, angiogenesis, and permeability of the BBB blood-brain barrier) [11]. In the brain, several DAMPs are reported to be released after an injury that leads to the activation of TLRs. Such DAMPs include Heat Shock Proteins, HMGB1, fibronectin, hyaluronic acid, nucleic acids such as mRNA and miRNAs, mitochondrial DNA, and N-formyl peptides [12 - 16]. Microglia express a full repertoire of TLRs in the brain, and microglial cells express mRNA for TLRs 1-9. Astrocytes also express TLRs 3,4, and 2 upon activation. Under resting and activating conditions astrocytes express TLR3. But TLR2 and 4 can be expressed upon activation only. Oligodendrocytes express both TLR2 and TLR3. Several TLRs can be expressed by neurons as well.TLR singaling through neurons is found to be involved in nociception. TLR4 can be seen as expressed in macrophages of CNS.

Cerebral Malaria and TLRs

It was long thought the brain is immunologically inert. The blood circulation in the brain also is supplied with T cells. These cells have been shown to experimentally sequester and activated in cerebral malaria during *Plasmodium berghei* infection. During experimental induction of Cerebral Malaria (CM), the sequestered αβ CD8 $^{+}$ T cells have a pathological effect [17, 18].

Further experimental studies on Cerebral Malaria, indicated specific proteins on Malaria induction in the brain such as PKC-θ signalling. This is very much essential for the recruitment of CD8(+) T cells to the brain thus resulting in pathological alterations of brain microvasculature. PKC-θ thus can be considered as one of the target molecules for CM [19] . Huggins *et al.*, 2017 [20] , have done a murine experimental CM, which showed CD8T cells, are responsible for

BBB breakdown. This BBB breakdown is associated with the reduction of claudin-5 and occuldins the tight junctional proteins.

Using TRIF-deficient mice it was shown that, in cerebral malaria, TLR 2 and TLR 9 mediated pathways in a MyD88-dependent manner have played a critical role in combating Pba infection [21]. Using Plamsmodium berghi model it is proven that the mice that are infected but deficient with TLR9 are not protected [22]. There are studies that point out that TLR7 deletion can protect against cerebral malaria in mice by altering cytokine production [23]. In Ugandan children, it was found that *TLR2* δ22 polymorphism is causing protection against cerebral malaria [24]. Experimental cerebral malaria is prevented by blocking the nucleic acid-sensing TLRs such as TLR9 [25]. Using meta-analysis it was shown that TLRs such as TLR1,4 and 9 are associated with high paracytemia and TLRs such as 2 and 6 are associated with the severity of the disease [26].

TLRs are synthesized in the endoplasmic reticulum, after which it goes to the Golgi apparatus. After some modification from Golgi apparatus either it goes to the plasma membrane or to the endosomes.The nucleic acid sensing TLRs are transported to the endosomes. Adaptors play an important role in the signaling of TLRs. There are various adaptors which are having TIR domains, these adaptors are recruited by various TLRs, the names of the adaptors are MyD88, TRIF, TIRAP/MAL, or TRAM. Myd88 is a common adaptor which is used by all the TLRs. Based on the usage of MyD88 TLR signaling pathways are divided as MyD88 dependent pathways and MyD88 independent pathways. In 1985, Toll gene was identified in drosophila by https://en.wikipedia.org/wiki/Christiane_N%C3%BCsslein-Volhard Christiane Nüsslein-Volhard. The study in drosophila has revealed that the gene that is involved in dorsoventral polarization is very similar to a gene that participates in innate immune signaling in the mammals. Due to this similarity the Toll is named after. In fruitfly embryos the toll pathways is very similar to mammalian IL-1R pathway indicating in fruitfly also Toll pathway can control the activities such as developmental patterning. The experiments with Toll mutant drosophila have revealed that the fly is not able to elicit immune responses against the fungal infections.

TLRs are transmemebrane proteins that contain 20–27, Extracellular Leucine-Rich Repeats (LRR). Each TLR can be recognized by their location, using of signal transduction molecules and signal transduction pathways. The MyD88 independent pathway is also called as TRIF pathways. Ubiquitination, phosphorylation and protein modifications play an important role in TLR mediated signaling. However, mutations in TLR signaling can lead to the development of various autoimmune diseases, and other inflammatory diseases.CD14 a co-receptor plays very important role in TLR signaling and proinflammatory signaling. For LPS recognition and other PAMPs recognition CD14 acts as a coreceptor along with MD14. TLRs signaling is also under the control of negative regulators as excessive activation of TLRs can lead to the over activation of immune system that producing various unwanted effects such as autoimmunity, allergies and inflammatory responses.

CONCLUDING REMARKS

Brain pericytes have been shown to express a variety of PRRS including TLRs, NOD and NLRs. There are 13 TLRs that are currently identified and all of them use Myd88 as their adaptor molecule except TLR3. It was long thought that the brain is immunologically inert. The blood circulation in the brain also is supplied with t cells. TLR-induced pathways can be bifurcated as two, based on their ability to use myeloid differentiation factor 88 (MyD88). Except for TLR3 all TLRs use the MyD88-dependent pathway, TLRs use the TRIF pathway to entice the inflammatory events. These PAMPs are recognised by PRRs and they have a pivotal role to play the infections and diseases by regulating chemokines and cytokines.

CONSENT FOR PUBLICATION

Not applicable.

CONFLICT OF INTEREST

The author declares no conflict of interest, financial or otherwise.

ACKNOWLEDGEMENT

Declared none.

REFERENCES

[1] Janeway CA Jr. The immune system evolved to discriminate infectious nonself from noninfectious self. Immunol Today 1992; 13(1): 11-6. [http://dx.doi.org/10.1016/0167-5699(92)90198-G] [PMID: 1739426]

[2] Matzinger P. Tolerance, danger, and the extended family. Annu Rev Immunol 1994; 12(1): 991-1045. [http://dx.doi.org/10.1146/annurev.iy.12.040194.005015] [PMID: 8011301]

[3] Alexopoulou L, Holt AC, Medzhitov R, Flavell RA. Recognition of double-stranded RNA and activation of NF-κB by Toll-like receptor 3. Nature 2001; 413(6857): 732-8. [http://dx.doi.org/10.1038/35099560] [PMID: 11607032]

[4] Poltorak A, He X, Smirnova I, Liu MY, Van Huffel C, Du X, *et al.* Defective LPS signaling in C3H/HeJ and C57BL/10ScCr mice: Mutations in TLR4 gene. Science (80-) 1998; 282(5396): 2085-8.

[5] Aliprantis AO, Yang RB, Mark MR, Suggett S, Devaux B, Radolf JD, *et al.* Cell activation and apoptosis by bacterial lipoproteins through toll- like receptor-2. Science (80-) 1999; 285(5428): 736-9.

[6] Temperley ND, Berlin S, Paton IR, Griffin DK, Burt DW. Evolution of the chicken Toll-like receptor gene family: A story of gene gain and gene loss. BMC Genomics 2008; 9(1): 62. [http://dx.doi.org/10.1186/1471-2164-9-62] [PMID: 18241342]

[7] Ciesielska A, Matyjek M, Kwiatkowska K. TLR4 and CD14 trafficking and its influence on LPS-induced pro-inflammatory signaling. Cell Mol Life Sci 2021; 78(4): 1233-61. [http://dx.doi.org/10.1007/s00018-020-03656-y] [PMID: 33057840]

[8] Gianni T, Campadelli-Fiume G. The epithelial αvβ3-integrin boosts the MYD88-dependent TLR2 signaling in response to viral and bacterial components. PLoS Pathog 2014; 10(11): e1004477. [http://dx.doi.org/10.1371/journal.ppat.1004477] [PMID: 25375272]

[9] Reuven EM, Fink A, Shai Y. Regulation of innate immune responses by transmembrane interactions: Lessons from the TLR family. Biochim Biophys Acta Biomembr 2014; 1838(6): 1586-93. [http://dx.doi.org/10.1016/j.bbamem.2014.01.020] [PMID: 24480409]

[10] Rustenhoven J, Jansson D, Smyth LC, Dragunow M. Brain pericytes as mediators of neuroinflammation. Trends Pharmacol Sci 2017; 38(3): 291-304. [http://dx.doi.org/10.1016/j.tips.2016.12.001] [PMID: 28017362]

[11] Sweeney MD, Ayyadurai S, Zlokovic BV. Pericytes of the neurovascular unit: Key functions and signaling pathways. Nat Neurosci 2016; 19(6): 771-83. [http://dx.doi.org/10.1038/nn.4288] [PMID: 27227366]

[12] Okamura Y, Watari M, Jerud ES, *et al.* The extra domain A of fibronectin activates Toll-like receptor 4. J Biol Chem 2001; 276(13): 10229-33. [http://dx.doi.org/10.1074/jbc.M100099200] [PMID: 11150311]

[13] Park JS, Svetkauskaite D, He Q, *et al.* Involvement of toll-like receptors 2 and 4 in cellular activation by high mobility group box 1 protein. J Biol Chem 2004; 279(9): 7370-7. [http://dx.doi.org/10.1074/jbc.M306793200] [PMID: 14660645]

[14] Li M, Carpio DF, Zheng Y, *et al.* An essential role of the NF-κ B/Toll-like receptor pathway in induction of inflammatory and tissue-repair gene expression by necrotic cells. J Immunol 2001; 166(12): 7128-35. [http://dx.doi.org/10.4049/jimmunol.166.12.7128] [PMID: 11390458]

[15] Karikó K, Ni H, Capodici J, Lamphier M, Weissman D. mRNA is an endogenous ligand for Toll-like receptor 3. J Biol Chem 2004; 279(13): 12542-50. [http://dx.doi.org/10.1074/jbc.M310175200] [PMID: 14729660]

[16] Liu JT, Lee IH, Wang CH, Chen KC, Lee CI, Yang YK. Cigarette smoking might impair memory and sleep quality. J Formos Med Assoc 2013; 112(5): 287-90. [http://dx.doi.org/10.1016/j.jfma.2011.12.006] [PMID: 23660225]

[17] Rénia L, Potter SM, Mauduit M, *et al.* Pathogenic T cells in cerebral malaria. Int J Parasitol 2006; 36(5): 547-54. [http://dx.doi.org/10.1016/j.ijpara.2006.02.007] [PMID: 16600241]

[18] Belnoue E, Kayibanda M, Vigario AM, *et al.* On the pathogenic role of brain-sequestered alphabeta CD8+ T cells in experimental cerebral malaria. J Immunol 2002; 169(11): 6369-75. [http://dx.doi.org/10.4049/jimmunol.169.11.6369] [PMID: 12444144]

[19] Fauconnier M, Bourigault ML, Meme S, *et al.* Protein kinase C-theta is required for development of experimental cerebral malaria. Am J Pathol 2011; 178(1): 212-21. [http://dx.doi.org/10.1016/j.ajpath.2010.11.008] [PMID: 21224058]

[20] Huggins MA, Johnson HL, Jin F, *et al.* Perforin expression by CD8 T cells is sufficient to cause fatal brain edema during experimental cerebral malaria. Infect Immun 2017; 85(5): 1-12. [http://dx.doi.org/10.1128/IAI.00985-16] [PMID: 28264905]

[21] Coban C, Ishii KJ, Uematsu S, *et al.* Pathological role of Toll-like receptor signaling in cerebral

malaria. Int Immunol 2006; 19(1): 67-79.
[http://dx.doi.org/10.1093/intimm/dxl123] [PMID: 17135446]

[22] Togbe D, Schofield L, Grau GE, *et al.* Murine cerebral malaria development is independent of toll-like receptor signaling. Am J Pathol 2007; 170(5): 1640-8.
[http://dx.doi.org/10.2353/ajpath.2007.060889] [PMID: 17456769]

[23] Baccarella A, Huang BW, Fontana MF, Kim CC. Loss of Toll-like receptor 7 alters cytokine production and protects against experimental cerebral malaria. Malar J 2014; 13(1): 354.
[http://dx.doi.org/10.1186/1475-2875-13-354] [PMID: 25192715]

[24] Greene JA, Sam-Agudu N, John CC, Opoka RO, Zimmerman PA, Kazura JW. Toll-like receptor polymorphisms and cerebral malaria: *TLR2* Δ22 polymorphism is associated with protection from cerebral malaria in a case control study. Malar J 2012; 11(1): 47.
[http://dx.doi.org/10.1186/1475-2875-11-47] [PMID: 22336003]

[25] Franklin BS, Ishizaka ST, Lamphier M, *et al.* Therapeutical targeting of nucleic acid-sensing Toll-like receptors prevents experimental cerebral malaria. Proc Natl Acad Sci USA 2011; 108(9): 3689-94.
[http://dx.doi.org/10.1073/pnas.1015406108] [PMID: 21303985]

[26] Ramirez Ramirez AD, de Jesus MCS, Rossit J, *et al.* Association of toll-like receptors in malaria susceptibility and immunopathogenesis: A meta-analysis. Heliyon 2022; 8(4): e09318.
[http://dx.doi.org/10.1016/j.heliyon.2022.e09318] [PMID: 35520620]

CHAPTER 3

Malaria

Abstract: The World Health Organization (WHO) defines cerebral malaria (CM) as an otherwise unexplained coma in a patient with asexual forms of malaria parasites on the peripheral blood smear. Malaria is a severe, devastating illness characterised by respiratory distress, severe anemia, and cerebral malaria (CM). Altered consciousness, convulsions, ataxia, hemiparesis, and other neurologic and psychiatric impairments are noted in cerebral malaria. Thus, cerebral malaria is defined as a condition in which a human has *Plasmodium falciparum*, a parasite in peripheral blood, followed by neurological complications of any degree. CM accounts for 300,000 deaths per year, and almost any survivors there display severe neurological manifestations. Coma is the outcome of CM, which is again due to brain hypoxia due to inflammation, edema, Brain swelling, and vascular blockage, are all due to the sequestration of pRBCs in brain microvasculature [1, 2]. In Ugandan children with CM infected with *P.falciparum*, severe cognitive impairment, behaviour problems such as hyperactivity, inattentiveness, aggressive behaviour, loss of speech, hearing loss, blindness, and epilepsy were noted (Irdo *et al.* , 2010). Heme offered protective responses to ECM, by dampening the activation of microglia, astrocytes, and expression of IP10, TNFa, and IFNg [3].

Keywords: Blood brain barrier (BBB), Glycosylphosphatidylinositol (GPI) anchors, *Plasmodium falciparum*, *Plasmodium berghei*, Postmalaria neurological syndrome (PMNS).

INTRODUCTION

MALARIA: PATHOLOGY IN THE BRAIN BY NEUROIMAGING

Malaria is the leading cause of death among infectious diseases globally. *Plasmodium falciparum* infection in children and adults causes cerebral malaria which is a primary cause of death in both groups [1]. Research on Cerebral Malaria (CM) is still elusive.

Both animal and human studies reveal various complicated features for the development of CM such as, increased pro-inflammatory cytokines, adhesion molecules, cytoadherence of parasite-infected erythrocytes, platelets, WBCs in the microvasculature of CNS [2 - 8].

Jayalakshmi Krishnan

Plasmodium falciparum infection in humans causes hearing loss in adults [8] and mental health disorders in children [2, 9 - 12]. Past evidence in people affected with cerebral malaria suggest that even after recovery they display brain injury in terms of cognitive deficits and neurological deficits in almost 25% of patients [9, 10, 12].

RBCs are parasitized (pRBCs), get adhere to the endothelium, and cause vasospasm. This is due to a reduced supply of Nitric Oxide. Once the blood vessel is blocked, it leads to the rupture of schizonts, leading to the accumulation of products of haemolysis. This in turn leads to more depletion of NO. All these mechanisms contribute to severe cerebral vasospasm. This further leads to brain swelling along with vaso-occulsion causing neuronal cell damage and death in CM [13].

Pathogenesis of cerebral malaria (CM), is conferred as microvascular obstruction, endothelial dysfunction, brain swelling, and impairment of blood-brain barrier, vasogenic edema, and venous congestion in both adults and children in Indian patients [13]. Basal nuclei consistency was also observed in MRI of patients suffering from CM. Further, studies also found in Patients that CM causes acute haemorrhagic infarctions were also seen in the brain stem, cerebellum, cerebral white matter, and insular cortex. This is followed by bithalamic infarctions with or without haemorrhages [14].

MRI in adults with severe *falciparum* malaria, revealed diffuse cerebral swelling, in adult Bangladeshi patients. These patients also showed focal extracellular oedema, cytotoxic oedema, and mildly raised brain lactate in MRI. In addition, these patients showed retinal whitening in patients with coma. However, subtle differences were noticed in children with cerebral edema in Malawian children, where severe effects of *falciparum* malaria were observed. Adult CM and coma are characterised by disturbances in microcirculation, and ischemia. This is attributed to sequestered parasites. These mechanisms can be taken into account for explaining the pathology of cerebral malaria in adults [15].

Plasmodium falciparum, the deadliest malarial parasite, kills 10 to 30% of people every year, it affects various organs of the body. Cytoadherence of parasite-infected erythrocytes in brain endothelium causes complications in CNS. Though adults and children both get the disease, the clinical manifestation and pathological occurrence entirely differ between the two groups, while coma remains a common symptom of both groups [16, 17]. On the other hand, in the case of the absence of severe or cerebral malaris in adults, MRI studies reveal acute cerebral injury with a lesion in the corpus callosum [18]. Cerebral venous sinus thrombosis is a complicated form of brain pathology in various infectious diseases, including malaria. Severe *falciparum* malaria resulted in increased intracranial pressure, and sinus thrombosis with venous infarction in a 43 old Thai patient [18].

Postmalaria neurological syndrome (PMNS), is reported to occur after two months of *falciparum* infection clearance. A 54-year-old Japanese man is reported to have PMNS with incoherent speech and disturbed and uncooperative behaviour with a high fever. Interestingly this patient displayed negative for malarial parasites in the Peripheral blood smear. Further, no organisms were found in CSF and MRI studies revealed no acute disseminated encephalomyelitis. Thus, PMNS remains an answered area of research [19]. Post cerebral malaria motor deficit is noted [20], and increased intracranial pressure followed by brain swelling is noted in children who died of malaria albeit not noted in survivors [21]. Comparative studies reveal in children with retinopathy-negative children display severe neurological deficits as observed by MRI in comparison with retinopathy-positive CM [22]. Atypical neurological manifestations were observed in patients infected with *P.falciparum* with cerebral venous thrombosis [21].

NOVEL MALARIA BIOMARKERS

Increased lactate and alanine concentrations are noted along with decreased aspartate and adenosine triphosphate levels which is due to hypoxia and ischemia whichin turn is due to clogged RBSc in brain microcirculation [2, 4]. interferon-γ, chemokine CXCL10, and lymphotoxin-α, in astrocytes, contribute to the development of cerebral malaria in murine as well as human primary astrocyte culture in experimental cerebral malaria [23]. Cerebral Malaria in children is also characterised by the high level of Osteoprotegrin (OPG), which is a protein stored in Weibel-Palade (WP) bodies. These are intracellular storage organelles in endothelial cells, during EC activation they get to fuse with the extracellular membrane and release their content. One such content is Osteoprotegrin (OPG), which is highly elevated in children with CM. Experimental cerebral malaria in mice has conformed to the elevated level of Osteoprotegrin (OPG), in mice [23]. Thus making it a new tool for malaria pathology. Thus identification of biomarkers for cerebral malaria becomes essential for therapeutic approaches. Apolipprotein E, present in the brain has been reported to be involved in various neurological diseases. The absence of Apoliproteptein E has protected the mouse brain from cerebral malaria, in which reduced T cell sequestration and parasites were seen [24]. Proteomic profiling of ECM, brains of C57/Bl6N mice infected with *P. berghei* ANKA has revealed potential biomarkers which could be the underlying cause of neurological manifestations [15].

BLOOD BRAIN BARRIER IN CEREBRAL MALARIA

Blood-brain barrier (BBB) is formed by astrocytes, pericytes, and endothelial cells. It regulates the flow of solutes between the CNS and blood. This is formed mainly by tight junctional proteins. Breakdown of BBB is noted in various neurodegenerative diseases, stress conditions, diseases, and insults to the brain [15]. *P. falciparum* secretes a unique protein called as Histidine-rich protein II (HRPII). The parasite makes the protein and transports it to the cytoplasm of RBC. Hemolysis of RBCs which are parasitized, emits the HRPII protein in the blood [25, 26].

Human cerebral microvascular endothelial cell line (hCMEC/D3) cells exposed to *P. falciparum* clone 3D7-parasitized erythrocytes showed disruption of the endothelial layer. Experiments *in vitro* have proven that clone Dd2, which contains a deletion of the HRPII gene, caused a minimal change in barrier integrity [27].

EXPERIMENTAL MOUSE MODELS FOR POTENTIAL TREATMENTS FOR HUMAN CM

How much are we Successful? *P.berghei* ANKA infection in CBA or CB57BL/6 mice is a widely used murine model to study experimental cerebral malaria. There are fundamental differences in the mechanisms of parasite sequestration by humans and mice. In mice, the leukocytes get parasites during an experimental CM, and then these cells get sequestered in the brain but in humans, which is a natural occurrence of the infection is characterised by intense intracerebral sequestration of parasitized RBCs in the Brain. So, extrapolation of the findings of the ECM to CM of humans is quite complicated as mice lacking WBCs may not catch up the ECM [28].

However, still a large number of publications are being done on experimental cerebral malaria. MRI studies in experimental murine CM reveal that BBB permeability was high in areas such as the lateral ventricle, olfactory bulb, and brainstem. Followed by brain swelling and edema. This effect was due to perforin, an effector molecule having a cytolytic effect, as inhibit studies in experimental CM reveal the protection from BBB leakage [3]. In experimental CM, mice infected with *Plasmodium berghei* ANKA (PbA) strain, MRI showed hippocampal abnormalities. Treatment of NMDA receptor antagonists reversed the changes, and offered neuroprotective effects in both the frontal cortex and hippocampus [29]. In experimental cerebral malaria, CD8+ T Cells are involved in brain pathology by inducing vascular breakage and neuronal death [29].

We are still a long way to developing an intervention based on the available data generated from experimental cerebral malaria. The immunopathological process plays a significant role in murine ECM, however, in human CM, it is the sequestered pRBCs in the endothelium, and the role of immune mechanisms is still elusive in the case of human CM. Secondly, in research on ECM, the mice can be taken into account before malaria, during malaria, and after malaria situations seldomly which is also possible with humans . A patient first comes with malaria to the hospital, and treatment with anti-malarial drugs is done followed by clinical investigations. Interventions based on the murine model are questionable here as in lad studies a controlled environment offers the expected results.

Knockout studies reveal that Irgm3-/- mice were shown to be protected from CM in cameraiton with Irgm1-/- mice. This protection of Irgm3-/- mice was due to less recruitment of CD8+ T cells within the brain and low production of inflammatory cytokines [5]. There are subtle differences in immune pathology of *Plasmodium berghei* ANKA (PbA) infected mice and P. yoelii 17XL (PyXL) infected mice, where the former develop cerebral malaria and later dies of parasitemia without neurological manifestations. Further studies on immunopathological changes reported that in ECM, pRBCs can be seen in the brain on three days of infection, tissue changes and edema on five days of infection followed by hemorrhage in different areas of the brain at the 7th day of infection [30]. It is interesting to note that even before BBB disruption, PbA-infected mice showed short-term memory impairment and spatial memory deficits. PbA-infection induced early short-term and spatial memory defects, prior to blood-brain barrier (BBB) disruption [30]. This was due to IL-33 receptor ST2, causing neurological inflammation and cognitive dysfunctions.

While the immuno pathological at ECM is highly investigated, the role of enzymes in accelerating or preventing ECM is still poorly understood. Some studies on this have shown that DUB cylindormatosis (CYLD), an enzyme that acts as an inhibitor of several cellular signalling pathways, is critically involved in promoting ECM. Knockout studies of *Cyld*$^{-/-}$ mice have survived the infection, whereas, congenic C57BL/6 mice, have shown disrupted BBB, enhanced parasite sequestration, *etc*. Interestingly, the sequestration of CD8 T cells, have reduced in ECM brain [31].

INHIBITOR STUDIES

Developing appropriate therapies for malaria remains a necessity. Often drug resistance, poor access to treatment, and the complexity of therapeutics made it complicated to treat malaria. Hence, studies on successful therapeutics thus become very essential. Recently, artesunate (AST) and recombinant human erythropoietin (rhEPO) have shown protective effects in the ECM model of C57BL/6 mice infected with *Plasmodium berghei* ANKA (PbA) by reducing CCL2, TNF-α, IFN-γ, IL-12, IL-18, CXCL9, and CXCL10, reduced endothelial activation, and protects blood-brain barrier [32].

DIAGNOSTIC AND THERAPEUTIC MONITORING OF CEREBRAL MALARIA BY IMAGING

Non-invasive methodology for early diagnosis of cerebral malaria would be a great task. Some studies in Experimental cerebral malaria throw light on liposomes containing indocyanine green (ICG) emissions in the infected and non-infected brain of ECM. The infected mice brain showed a greater emission in comparison with the non-infected one. The emission was further confined by histopathological studies which revealed the presence of liposomal ICG in areas where phagocytes have taken up the dye [31]. Sometimes, structural imaging like CT and MRI may not provide accurate things, there is a chance to see non-specific information. SPECT perfusion is used nowadays to monitor Cerebral malaria in humans [31].

MALARIA AND TOLL-LIKE RECEPTORS IN THE BRAIN

Toll-like receptor 9 has been targeted by chloroquine (CQ) to ameliorate the experimental cerebral malaria in C57BL/6 mice upon infection by *P.berghei* ANKA (PbA) (Zhu *et al.* , 2012). Various cytokines act differently in various disease situations. TLR7 agonist imidazoquinoline (BBIQ) treatment along with CQ against *P. berghei* ANKA (PbA) in mice has shown that the inflammatory T cells in the brain of the mice were lower. On the other hand, the serum levels of IFN-γ and IL-12 were higher in the mice suggesting a strong TH1 response against the parasite by BBIQ and CQ treatment [31]. Thus the agonist of TLRs which is immunomodulatory in nature can give effective results when combined with CQ. TLR9, TLR7, TLR4, and TLR2 have been shown to play an important role in the pathogenesis of severe cerebral and other forms of malaria [33 - 35].

Plasmodium antigens can activate TLR2, TLR4, and TLR9, and most recently also TLR7. A study found that Glycosylphosphatidylinositol (GPI) anchors in a higher purification state from T. cruzi parasites activate the TLR2 immune responses [36]. This kind of immune activation may lead to a defence mechanism for the evasion of any protozoan parasite. MyD88, TLR2, and TLR9 KO mice have shown there is resistance to the *P.berghi* infection in the brain by reducing the brain leukocyte infiltration and cytokine production [37, 38]. Mice lacking TLR9 is not been scavenged from CM, displaying microvascular damage and leak in the brain [39]. TLR2 has been shown to bind with glycosylphosphatidylinositol

(GPI) from *P. falciparum*-and any mutations in the TLR2 gene may cause the disease prognosis to worsen [40]. TLR7 deletion has been associated with partial protection from experimental cerebral malaria and also promoted more anti-inflammatory cytokine production.

Experimental cerebral malaria is prevented by targeting human or mouse TLR9 with synthetic antagonists such as E6446 [41]. In MyD88 deficient mice, Hemozoin load and parasitic sequestration were lesser in comparison with WT mice upon *Plasmodium berghei* ANKA (PbA) infection [37, 38, 38]. Rodent model Malaria parasite caused increased TLR responses which are dependent on IFNɣ [41]. Natural infection with *P.falciparum* in humans has shown the elevation of TLR responses. TLR2, TLR3 and TLR4 have been shown to respond to GPI from *P.falciparum* whereas hemozoin is detected by TLR9 [42]. Mice immunised with GPI upon infection with *Plasmodium berghi* have shown better protection from acidosis and pulmonary edema in comparison with non-immunized mice [39, 43, 44]. Hemozoin is a detoxification product generated in the food vacuoles of *Plasmodium* parasite [45, 46] and TLR9 causes innate immune responses by Hemozoin [37, 38]. Hemozoin induces direct inflammatory responses by binding to TLR9 which is an endosomal receptor [47].

TLR polymorphisms are known to be either resistant or susceptibile to infections by *Plasmodium.* Variants of TLR1 and 6 tied up with mild malaria symptoms whereas high parasitemia is caused by *TLR-9-1486C/T* variants [48]. Also, *TLR-9 -1486C/T* (rs1870884) is involved in placental malaria [49]. TLR9 is the most investigated receptor for polymorphism studies. Different polymorphisms of TLRs show different kinds of responses to various malaria parasites in different places.

Some reports say that during the liver stage of infection, *plasmodium* RNA acts as a malaria parasitic ligand [49]. A recent study during the molecular docking method study points out that glycosylphosphatidylinositols (GPIs) from *Plasmodium falciparum* binding mode is very similar to the lipopeptides, thus suggesting the lipid areas of both the ligands can mediate the dimerization of TLR2 receptors [49]. All the ligands of the malaria parasite that bind with TLRs are given in Table **1**. Polymorphisms that enhance malaria disease are shown in Table **2**.

Table 1. TLR ligands and their receptors of Malaria parasite.

Type of TLR Receptor	Ligand	References
TLR2 with TLR1 or TLR6 heterodimer	*P. falciparum* glycosylphosphatidylinositol (GPI)	Krishnegowda *et al.* , 2005 [42]
TLR4	*P. falciparum* glycosylphosphatidylinositol (GPI)	Krishnegowda *et al.* , 2005 [41]
TLR 9	*Plasmodium* DNA	Parroche *et al.* , 2007 [47]
TLR2 TLR9	Hz	Coban *et al.* , 2005 [50] Coban *et al.* , 2007
TLR-4 and CD11b/CD18-integrin	Host fibrinogen stably bound to hemozoin	Barrera V *et al.* , 2011 [50]

Table 2. TLR polymorphism in Malaria.

TLR	*SNPs*	-	-
TLR-1	S248N	placental malaria	Hamann, *et al.* , 2010 [49, 51]
TLR-4	-	-	-
TLR-6--249P allele	*S249P* SNP	risk factor for malaria	Fabiana *et al.* ,2008 [48]
TLR-9	T1237C rs5743836	symptomatic malaria/ higher mean parasitaemia	*Omar et al.* , 2012 [52]
TLR-9-1486C allele	*1486C/T*	high parasitemia	Fabiana *et al.* , 2008 [48]

TLR 9 (T1486C and T1237C) polymorphisms are known to be involved in malaria progression in some geographical areas [53]. Upon *plasmodium* infection, MyD88-/- mice showed less cytokine production [54, 55]. Innate immune responses through TLRs are enhanced in the PBMSc of patients with malaria infection [56]. *Plasmodium* strains cause innate immune responses by activating the interleukins and interferons upon *plasmodium* infection through TLR7 [57]. In BALB/c mice also these findings are extended that for blood-stage *Plasmodium chabaudi* infection in dendrite cells, TH1 cells, and T Reg cells treated with agonists of TLR4, 7 and 9 have enhanced immune responses [58]. *Plasmodium yoelii (Py)* infection with cells of DBA/2 mouse through TLR 4 and 9 has shown protective responses by resisting the malaria parasites [59]. *Plasmodium yoelii* infection with mice lacking various TLRs and MyD88, TLR9, and MyD88 are essential for regulating immune responses against the parasite [60]. *Plasmodium yoelii* 17XNL infection with BALB/c mice upregulated MyD88, TRF6, IRAK1 and TLR2 [61]. In Amazonas, Brazil a study was conducted in which it was found that for *Plasmodium vivax*-induced infection TLR5 R392StopCodon and TLR9 -1486C/T variants were involved [62]. In the same area of study, it was found that cytokine levels were changed due to SNPs in

various TLRs [63]. Upon infection with *Plasmodium yoelii*, TLR2 signaling yields significant suppression of the parasite development, in TLR2 and MyD88 -/- mice, there was a higher parasitemia and liver parasitic load [64]. There are studies on TLR polymorphisms and birth weight in infants when the mother is infected with the malaria parasite. These studies indicated that TLR4 and TLR9 polymorphisms are associated with low birth weight in pregnant women exposed to malaria parasites [65]. In a recombinant *Mycobacterium bovis* bacille Calmette-Guérin (rBCG) expressing C-terminus of merozoite surface protein-1, from mice infected with *P.falciparum*, it is observed thattoll-like receptors causes expression of various immunoglobulin's, and interleukins [66].

MALARIA DRUGS AND MECHANISM OF ACTION

Antimalarial drugs such as chloroquine, quinine and mefloquine, are used against the malaria parasite. Chloroquine is an aminoquinolone derivative and it destroys the food vacuole of the parasite, and also other drugs act at the blood stages of the parasite. *Plasmodium falciparaum* is chloroquine sensitive and this rug can be used against it. Chloroquine Phosphate can be used to treat uncomplicated malaria. Hydroxychloroquine can be used to with same sensitivity as like Chloroquine Phosphate as first line of treatment [67, 68]. For treatment to P. vivax or P. ovale infections primaquine phosphate is used as an additional agent along with other drugs [69]. For parasites with chloroquine resistance artemether-lumefantrine and atovaquone-proguanil is used. For treating severe malaria cases along with firs tline of treatment with quinine drugs Doxycycline, Clindamycin, Tetracycline should also be used. For the treatment of malaria chloroquine was developed in 1940s, until the development of novel antimalarial drugs such as mefloquine, artemisnin and pyrimethamine. Chroloroquine is not only for the treatment of malaria it is also used to treat other diseases such as rheumatoid arthritis, HIV and systemic lupus erythematosus. Artemether is the antimalarial drug which is designed at targeting the erythrocytic stages *P.falciparum*. This drug actually inhibits the nucleic acid and prevents protein synthesis. The action of this drug is through by inhibiting the beta hematin formation and endoperoxide creation.

CONCLUDING REMARKS

Ligands from the malaria parasite can be classified as blood-stage parasitic ligands and liver-stage parasitic ligands, the research on the ligands and their binding nature with various TLRs are very scanty. Research being conducted in the human form of CM has posted various questions thsat can we develop a model to study human cerebral malaria by mimicking the mouse model.

CONSENT FOR PUBLICATION

Not applicable.

CONFLICT OF INTEREST

The author declares no conflict of interest, financial or otherwise.

ACKNOWLEDGEMENT

Declared none.

REFERENCES

[1] Menezes RG, Pant S, Kharoshah MA, *et al.* Autopsy discoveries of death from malaria. Leg Med (Tokyo) 2012; 14(3): 111-5. [http://dx.doi.org/10.1016/j.legalmed.2012.01.007] [PMID: 22369777]

[2] Idro R, Marsh K, John CC, Newton CRJ. Cerebral malaria: mechanisms of brain injury and strategies for improved neurocognitive outcome. Pediatr Res 2010; 68(4): 267-74. [http://dx.doi.org/10.1203/PDR.0b013e3181eee738] [PMID: 20606600]

[3] Huggins MA, Johnson HL, Jin F, *et al.* Perforin expression by CD8 T cells is sufficient to cause fatal brain edema during experimental cerebral malaria. Infect Immun 2017; 85(5): 1-12. [http://dx.doi.org/10.1128/IAI.00985-16] [PMID: 28264905]

[4] Miller LH, Baruch DI, Marsh K, Doumbo OK. The pathogenic basis of malaria. Nature 2002; 415(6872): 673-9. [http://dx.doi.org/10.1038/415673a] [PMID: 11832955]

[5] Guo J, McQuillan JA, Yau B, *et al.* IRGM3 contributes to immunopathology and is required for differentiation of antigen-specific effector CD8+ T cells in experimental cerebral malaria. Infect Immun 2015; 83(4): 1406-17. [http://dx.doi.org/10.1128/IAI.02701-14] [PMID: 25644000]

[6] Swanson PA II, Hart GT, Russo MV, *et al.* CD8+ T cells induce fatal brainstem pathology during cerebral malaria *via* luminal antigen-specific engagement of brain vasculature. PLoS Pathog 2016; 12(12): e1006022. [http://dx.doi.org/10.1371/journal.ppat.1006022] [PMID: 27907215]

[7] Kwiatkowski D, Sambou I, Twumasi P, *et al.* TNF concentration in fatal cerebral, non-fatal cerebral, and uncomplicated *Plasmodium falciparum* malaria. Lancet 1990; 336(8725): 1201-4. [http://dx.doi.org/10.1016/0140-6736(90)92827-5] [PMID: 1978068]

[8] Kern P, Hemmer CJ, Damme JV, Gruss HJ, Dietrich M. Elevated tumor necrosis factor alpha and interleukin-6 serum levels as markers for complicated *plasmodium falciparum* malaria. Am J Med 1989; 87(2): 139-43. [http://dx.doi.org/10.1016/S0002-9343(89)80688-6] [PMID: 2667356]

[9] Idro R, Kakooza-Mwesige A, Balyejjussa S, *et al.* Severe neurological sequelae and behaviour problems after cerebral malaria in Ugandan children. BMC Res Notes 2010; 3(1): 104. [http://dx.doi.org/10.1186/1756-0500-3-104] [PMID: 20398391]

[10] John CC, Bangirana P, Byarugaba J, *et al.* Cerebral malaria in children is associated with long-term cognitive impairment. Pediatrics 2008; 122(1): e92-9. [http://dx.doi.org/10.1542/peds.2007-3709] [PMID: 18541616]

[11] Idro R, Carter JA, Fegan G, Neville BGR, Newton CRJC. Risk factors for persisting neurological and cognitive impairments following cerebral malaria. Arch Dis Child 2005; 91(2): 142-8.

[http://dx.doi.org/10.1136/adc.2005.077784] [PMID: 16326798]

[12] Idro R, Jenkins NE, Newton CRJC. Pathogenesis, clinical features, and neurological outcome of cerebral malaria. Lancet Neurol 2005; 4(12): 827-40.
[http://dx.doi.org/10.1016/S1474-4422(05)70247-7] [PMID: 16297841]

[13] Eisenhut M. The evidence for a role of vasospasm in the pathogenesis of cerebral malaria. Malar J 2015; 14(1): 405.
[http://dx.doi.org/10.1186/s12936-015-0928-4] [PMID: 26463364]

[14] Rasalkar DD, Paunipagar BK, Sanghvi D, Sonawane BD, Loniker P. Magnetic resonance imaging in cerebral malaria: a report of four cases. Br J Radiol 2011; 84(1000): 380-5.
[http://dx.doi.org/10.1259/bjr/85759874] [PMID: 21415303]

[15] Moussa E, Huang H, Ahras M, *et al.* Proteomic profiling of the brain of mice with experimental cerebral malaria. J Proteomics 2018; 180(2): 61-9.
[http://dx.doi.org/10.1016/j.jprot.2017.06.002] [PMID: 28602553]

[16] Haldar K, Murphy SC, Milner DA Jr, Taylor TE. Malaria: mechanisms of erythrocytic infection and pathological correlates of severe disease. Annu Rev Pathol 2007; 2(1): 217-49.
[http://dx.doi.org/10.1146/annurev.pathol.2.010506.091913] [PMID: 18039099]

[17] Dondorp AM, Lee SJ, Faiz MA, *et al.* The relationship between age and the manifestations of and mortality associated with severe malaria. Clin Infect Dis 2008; 47(2): 151-7.
[http://dx.doi.org/10.1086/589287] [PMID: 18533842]

[18] Luvira V, Chamnanchanunt S, Thanachartwet V, Phumratanaprapin W, Viriyavejakul A. Cerebral venous sinus thrombosis in severe malaria. Southeast Asian J Trop Med Public Health 2009; 40(5): 893-7.
[PMID: 19842369]

[19] Mizuno Y, Kato Y, Kanagawa S, *et al.* A case of postmalaria neurological syndrome in Japan. J Infect Chemother 2006; 12(6): 399-401.
[http://dx.doi.org/10.1016/S1341-321X(06)70902-3] [PMID: 17235648]

[20] Taiaa O, Amil T, Darbi A. Hemiparesis post cerebral malaria. Pan Afr Med J 2015; 20(1): 1-8.
[PMID: 25995798]

[21] Michie HR, Manogue KR, Spriggs DR, *et al.* Detection of circulating tumor necrosis factor after endotoxin administration. N Engl J Med 1988; 318(23): 1481-6.
[http://dx.doi.org/10.1056/NEJM198806093182301] [PMID: 2835680]

[22] Postels DG, Taylor TE, Kampondeni SD, *et al.* Brain MRI of children with retinopathy-negative cerebral malaria. Am J Trop Med Hyg 2014; 91(5): 943-9.
[http://dx.doi.org/10.4269/ajtmh.14-0216] [PMID: 25200262]

[23] Bakmiwewa SM, Weiser S, Grey M, *et al.* Synergistic induction of CXCL10 by interferon-gamma and lymphotoxin-alpha in astrocytes: Possible role in cerebral malaria. Cytokine 2016; 78(1): 79-86.
[http://dx.doi.org/10.1016/j.cyto.2015.11.024] [PMID: 26687629]

[24] Kassa FA, Van Den Ham K, Rainone A, Fournier S, Boilard E, Olivier M. Absence of apolipoprotein E protects mice from cerebral malaria. Sci Rep 2016; 6(1): 33615.
[http://dx.doi.org/10.1038/srep33615] [PMID: 27647324]

[25] Wellems TE, Howard RJ. Homologous genes encode two distinct histidine-rich proteins in a cloned isolate of *Plasmodium falciparum*. Proc Natl Acad Sci USA 1986; 83(16): 6065-9.
[http://dx.doi.org/10.1073/pnas.83.16.6065] [PMID: 3016741]

[26] Howard G, Wagenknecht LE, Cai J, Cooper L, Kraut MA, Toole JF. Cigarette smoking and other risk factors for silent cerebral infarction in the general population. Stroke 1998; 29(5): 913-7.
[http://dx.doi.org/10.1161/01.STR.29.5.913] [PMID: 9596234]

[27] Pal P, Daniels BP, Oskman A, Diamond MS, Klein RS, Goldberg DE. *Plasmodium falciparum*

histidine-rich protein II compromises brain endothelial barriers and may promote cerebral malaria pathogenesis. MBio 2016; 7(3): e00617-16.
[http://dx.doi.org/10.1128/mBio.00617-16] [PMID: 27273825]

[28] White NJ, Turner GDH, Medana IM, Dondorp AM, Day NPJ. The murine cerebral malaria phenomenon. Trends Parasitol 2010; 26(1): 11-5.
[http://dx.doi.org/10.1016/j.pt.2009.10.007] [PMID: 19932638]

[29] de Miranda AS, Brant F, Vieira LB, *et al.* A Neuroprotective Effect of the Glutamate Receptor Antagonist MK801 on Long-Term Cognitive and Behavioral Outcomes Secondary to Experimental Cerebral Malaria. Mol Neurobiol 2017; 54(9): 7063-82.
[http://dx.doi.org/10.1007/s12035-016-0226-3] [PMID: 27796746]

[30] Khandare AV, Bobade D, Deval M, Patil T, Saha B, Prakash D. Expression of negative immune regulatory molecules, pro-inflammatory chemokine and cytokines in immunopathology of ECM developing mice. Acta Trop 2017; 172(20): 58-63.
[http://dx.doi.org/10.1016/j.actatropica.2017.04.025] [PMID: 28454880]

[31] Portnoy E, Vakruk N, Bishara A, *et al.* Indocyanine Green Liposomes for Diagnosis and Therapeutic Monitoring of Cerebral Malaria. Theranostics 2016; 6(2): 167-76.
[http://dx.doi.org/10.7150/thno.13653] [PMID: 26877776]

[32] Du Y, Chen G, Zhang X, Yu C, Cao Y, Cui L. Artesunate and erythropoietin synergistically improve the outcome of experimental cerebral malaria. Int Immunopharmacol 2017; 48(18): 219-30.
[http://dx.doi.org/10.1016/j.intimp.2017.05.008] [PMID: 28531845]

[33] Gazzinelli RT, Kalantari P, Fitzgerald KA, Golenbock DT. Innate sensing of malaria parasites. Nat Rev Immunol 2014; 14(11): 744-57.
[http://dx.doi.org/10.1038/nri3742] [PMID: 25324127]

[34] Olivier M, Van Den Ham K, Shio MT, Kassa FA, Fougeray S. Malarial pigment hemozoin and the innate inflammatory response. Front Immunol 2014; 5(FEB): 25.
[http://dx.doi.org/10.3389/fimmu.2014.00025] [PMID: 24550911]

[35] M Eriksson E. Toll-like receptors and malaria – sensing and susceptibility. J Trop Dis 2014; 02(01): 1-7.

[36] Campos MAS, Almeida IC, Takeuchi O, *et al.* Activation of Toll-like receptor-2 by glycosylphosphatidylinositol anchors from a protozoan parasite. J Immunol 2001; 167(1): 416-23.
[http://dx.doi.org/10.4049/jimmunol.167.1.416] [PMID: 11418678]

[37] Coban C, Ishii KJ, Kawai T, *et al.* Toll-like receptor 9 mediates innate immune activation by the malaria pigment hemozoin. J Exp Med 2005; 201(1): 19-25.
[http://dx.doi.org/10.1084/jem.20041836] [PMID: 15630134]

[38] Coban C, Ishii KJ, Uematsu S, *et al.* Pathological role of Toll-like receptor signaling in cerebral malaria. Int Immunol 2006; 19(1): 67-79.
[http://dx.doi.org/10.1093/intimm/dxl123] [PMID: 17135446]

[39] Togbe D, Schofield L, Grau GE, *et al.* Murine cerebral malaria development is independent of toll-like receptor signaling. Am J Pathol 2007; 170(5): 1640-8.
[http://dx.doi.org/10.2353/ajpath.2007.060889] [PMID: 17456769]

[40] Greene JA, Sam-Agudu N, John CC, Opoka RO, Zimmerman PA, Kazura JW. Toll-like receptor polymorphisms and cerebral malaria: TLR2 Δ22 polymorphism is associated with protection from cerebral malaria in a case control study. Malar J 2012; 11(1): 47.
[http://dx.doi.org/10.1186/1475-2875-11-47] [PMID: 22336003]

[41] Franklin BS, Ishizaka ST, Lamphier M, *et al.* Therapeutical targeting of nucleic acid-sensing Toll-like receptors prevents experimental cerebral malaria. Proc Natl Acad Sci USA 2011; 108(9): 3689-94.
[http://dx.doi.org/10.1073/pnas.1015406108] [PMID: 21303985]

[42] Krishnegowda G, Hajjar AM, Zhu J, *et al.* Induction of proinflammatory responses in macrophages by

the glycosylphosphatidylinositols of *Plasmodium falciparum*: cell signaling receptors, glycosylphosphatidylinositol (GPI) structural requirement, and regulation of GPI activity. J Biol Chem 2005; 280(9): 8606-16.
[http://dx.doi.org/10.1074/jbc.M413541200] [PMID: 15623512]

[43] Schofield L, Hewitt MC, Evans K, Siomos MA, Seeberger PH. Synthetic GPI as a candidate anti-toxic vaccine in a model of malaria. Nature 2002; 418(6899): 785-9.
[http://dx.doi.org/10.1038/nature00937] [PMID: 12181569]

[44] Schofield L, Grau GE. Immunological processes in malaria pathogenesis. Nat Rev Immunol 2005; 5(9): 722-35.
[http://dx.doi.org/10.1038/nri1686] [PMID: 16138104]

[45] Sullivan DJ. Theories on malarial pigment formation and quinoline action. Int J Parasitol 2002; 32(13): 1645-53.
[http://dx.doi.org/10.1016/S0020-7519(02)00193-5] [PMID: 12435449]

[46] Arese P, Schwarzer E. Malarial pigment (haemozoin): a very active 'inert' substance. Ann Trop Med Parasitol 1997; 91(5): 501-16.
[http://dx.doi.org/10.1080/00034983.1997.11813168] [PMID: 9329987]

[47] Parroche P, Lauw FN, Goutagny N, *et al.* Malaria hemozoin is immunologically inert but radically enhances innate responses by presenting malaria DNA to Toll-like receptor 9. Proc Natl Acad Sci USA 2007; 104(6): 1919-24.
[http://dx.doi.org/10.1073/pnas.0608745104] [PMID: 17261807]

[48] Leoratti FMS, Farias L, Alves FP, *et al.* Variants in the toll-like receptor signaling pathway and clinical outcomes of malaria. J Infect Dis 2008; 198(5): 772-80.
[http://dx.doi.org/10.1086/590440] [PMID: 18662133]

[49] Henningfield J, Cohen C, Pickworth W. Psychopharmacology of nicotine 1993; 25-45.

[50] Hamann L, Bedu-Addo G, Eggelte TA, Schumann RR, Mockenhaupt FP. The toll-like receptor 1 variant S248N influences placental malaria. Infect Genet Evol 2010; 10(6): 785-9.
[http://dx.doi.org/10.1016/j.meegid.2010.05.005] [PMID: 20478407]

[51] Omar AH, Yasunami M, Yamazaki A, *et al.* Toll-like receptor 9 (TLR9) polymorphism associated with symptomatic malaria: a cohort study. Malar J 2012; 11(1): 168.
[http://dx.doi.org/10.1186/1475-2875-11-168] [PMID: 22594374]

[52] Naing C, Wong ST, Aung HH. Toll-like receptor 9 and 4 gene polymorphisms in susceptibility and severity of malaria: a meta-analysis of genetic association studies. Malar J 2021; 20(1): 302.
[http://dx.doi.org/10.1186/s12936-021-03836-6] [PMID: 34217314]

[53] Franklin BS, Rodrigues SO, Antonelli LR, *et al.* MyD88-dependent activation of dendritic cells and CD4+ T lymphocytes mediates symptoms, but is not required for the immunological control of parasites during rodent malaria. Microbes Infect 2007; 9(7): 881-90.
[http://dx.doi.org/10.1016/j.micinf.2007.03.007] [PMID: 17537666]

[54] Adachi K, Tsutsui H, Kashiwamura SI, *et al. Plasmodium berghei* infection in mice induces liver injury by an IL-12- and toll-like receptor/myeloid differentiation factor 88-dependent mechanism. J Immunol 2001; 167(10): 5928-34.
[http://dx.doi.org/10.4049/jimmunol.167.10.5928] [PMID: 11698470]

[55] McCall MBB, Netea MG, Hermsen CC, *et al. Plasmodium falciparum* infection causes proinflammatory priming of human TLR responses. J Immunol 2007; 179(1): 162-71.
[http://dx.doi.org/10.4049/jimmunol.179.1.162] [PMID: 17579034]

[56] Baccarella A, Fontana MF, Chen EC, Kim CC. Toll-like receptor 7 mediates early innate immune responses to malaria. Infect Immun 2013; 81(12): 4431-42.
[http://dx.doi.org/10.1128/IAI.00923-13] [PMID: 24042114]

[57] Gao W, Sun X, Li D, *et al.* Toll-like receptor 4, Toll-like receptor 7 and Toll-like receptor 9 agonists

enhance immune responses against blood-stage *Plasmodium chabaudi* infection in BALB/c mice. Int Immunopharmacol 2020; 89(Pt B): 107096.
[http://dx.doi.org/10.1016/j.intimp.2020.107096]

[58] Zhang Y, Zhu X, Feng Y, *et al.* Toll-like receptor 4, Toll-like receptor 7 and Toll-like receptor 9 agonists enhance immune responses against blood-stage *Plasmodium chabaudi* infection in BALB/c mice. Int Immunopharmacol. Exp Parasitol 2016; 170: 73-81.
[http://dx.doi.org/10.1016/j.exppara.2016.09.003] [PMID: 27646627]

[59] Gowda NM, Wu X, Gowda DC. TLR9 and MyD88 are crucial for the development of protective immunity to malaria. J Immunol 2012; 188(10): 5073-85.
[http://dx.doi.org/10.4049/jimmunol.1102143] [PMID: 22516959]

[60] Fu Y, Ding Y, Zhou T, Fu X, Xu W. *Plasmodium yoelii* blood-stage primes macrophage-mediated innate immune response through modulation of toll-like receptor signalling. Malar J 2012; 11(1): 104.
[http://dx.doi.org/10.1186/1475-2875-11-104] [PMID: 22463100]

[61] Costa AG, Ramasawmy R, Ibiapina HNS, *et al.* Association of TLR variants with susceptibility to *Plasmodium vivax* malaria and parasitemia in the Amazon region of Brazil. PLoS One 2017; 12(8): e0183840.
[http://dx.doi.org/10.1371/journal.pone.0183840] [PMID: 28850598]

[62] Costa AG, Ramasawmy R, Val FFA, *et al.* Polymorphisms in TLRs influence circulating cytokines production in *Plasmodium vivax* malaria. Cytokine 2018; 110: 374-80.
[http://dx.doi.org/10.1016/j.cyto.2018.04.008] [PMID: 29656958]

[63] Zheng H, Tan Z, Zhou T, *et al.* The TLR2 is activated by sporozoites and suppresses intrahepatic rodent malaria parasite development. Sci Rep 2015; 5(1): 18239.
[http://dx.doi.org/10.1038/srep18239] [PMID: 26667391]

[64] Mockenhaupt FP, Hamann L, von Gaertner C, *et al.* Common polymorphisms of toll-like receptors 4 and 9 are associated with the clinical manifestation of malaria during pregnancy. J Infect Dis 2006; 194(2): 184-8.
[http://dx.doi.org/10.1086/505152] [PMID: 16779724]

[65] Abbas and Subian. Role of toll-like receptor 4 in eliciting adaptive immune responses against recombinant BCG expressing the C-terminus of merozoite surface protein-1 of *Plasmodium falciparum*. Parasitological research 2019; 9(1): 40-6.

[66] NAß J, Efferth T. The activity of artemisia spp. and their constituents against trypanosomiasis. phytomedicine. 2018 Aug 01;47: 184-191.

[67] Pinheiro LCS, FEITOSA LM, Silveira FFD, Boechat N. Current antimalarial therapies and advances in the development of semi-synthetic artemisinin derivatives. An acad bras cienc. 2018; 90(1 Suppl 2): 1251-1271.

[68] Karunajeewa H, James R. Primaquine for *Plasmodium vivax* malaria treatment. Lancet. 2020 Jun 27; 395(10242): 1971-1972.

[69] Hama luba M, van der Pluijm RW, Weya J, *et al.* Arterolane-piperaquine-mefloquine versus arterolane-piperaquine and artemether-lumefantrine in the treatment of uncomplicated *Plasmodium falciparum* malaria in Kenyan children: a single-centre, open-label, randomised, non-inferiority trial. Lancet Infect Dis. 2021 21(10): 1395-1406.

CHAPTER 4

TLRs in Lymphatic Filariasis

Abstract: Lymphatic filariasis is one of the neglected tropical diseases and also a disfiguring vector-borne disease. Parasitic nematodes such as *Wuchereriabancrofti*, *Brugiamalayi*, and *Brugiatimori* are the three types of parasites that cause lymphatic pathology in terms of *hydrocele, lymphedema, and elephantiasis* [1]. Among these three parasites, *Wuchereriabancrofti* is the principal parasite, which causes around 90% of infections. These nematodes impair the lymphatic system, thus leading to considerable morbidity in the affected people. The life cycle of this adult-stage lymph-dwelling parasites is complex in nature. Once they start infecting the lymphatics, they cause swelling, dilatation, and thickening of lymph vessels.

Keywords: Bancroftian filariasis, *B. malayi*, Proinflammatory cytokines, *Wolbachia* lipoproteins, *Wuchereria bancrofti.*

INTRODUCTION

Immune cell interaction with a parasite is of paramount importance as they could just lead to immunopathogenesis. Dendritic cells are known as antigen-presenting cells as they can mount the T cell-derived immune responses.

The sheath antigen protein which is of 70kDa from *Wuchereriabancrofti* binds with the human dendritic cells and causes the maturation of the cells along with proinflammatory cytokine secretion *via* toll-like receptor 4 signaling [1, 2]. TLR polymorphisms are involved in making the disease susceptible to the pathogen. TLR 2 -196 to -173 polymorphism in the 5' untranslated region is reported from the blood samples collected from the Tanga region with bancroftianfilariasis [3]. Unlike viral and bacterial infections filarial infections cause immunomodulation, for example, it has been shown that pre-infection with filarial parasites, protects the mice from both types of diabetes [4]. In line with these studies, filariasis, and *Mycobacterium tuberculosis* confection studies also have shown that filarial antigens cause immunomodulation by inhibiting the TLR2 and TLR9 expression [4]. *Wolbachia* is a symbiotic bacteria living inside the filarial nematode and WSP (Wolbachia Surface protein) from these species induces a strong inflammatory process through TLR2 and TLR4 in dendritic cells and macrophages [5]. There are studies that point out that *Wolbachia* lipoproteins augment the immune respo-

Jayalakshmi Krishnan

nse to *B. malayi* by stimulating both innate and adaptive immune response through TLR2 and 6 [6]. Diminished TLR (TLR1, TLR2, TLR4, and TLR9) expression is seen in macrophages during filarial infection but not in monocytes [7]. Lacto-N-fucopentose III (LNFPIII)and phosphorylcholine-decorated glycans from filarial parasite act as pattern recognition receptors to TLR4 [8]. MF-exposed monocyte-derived human DCs (mhDCs) showed decreased expression of TLR4 and TLR3 mRNA in comparison with unexposed cells [7]. T cell expression of TLR9 was not diminished during the filarial infection but TLR1, TLR2, and TLR4 expression was lowered [8]. Filarial antigen from Brugiapahangi (BpA) triggers apoptosis of normal human monocytes through TLR 4 [8].

Proinflammatory cytokines are the key inducers of lymphatic filariasis-induced pathology. Attempts have been made to understand the impact of lymphatic filariasis in triggering the TLRs. Cytokine responses in patients of chronic, subclinical pathology and uninfected; individuals have shown that TLR2,7 and TLR 9n mediated inflammatory responses were higher in the chronically infected group [8]. This response is mediated by extracellular signal-regulated kinase 1/2 (ERK1/2) and p38 mitogen-activated protein (MAP) kinases (MAPK) hyperphosphorylation. NF-κB also hyperphosphorylated in chronically infected individuals. In Thailand, an investigation of SNPs was found to be associated with TLR2 −196 to −173 del, +597 T>C, and +1350 T>C polymorphisms in asymptomatic bancroftian filariasis [9].

When the discovery of endosymbiotic *Wolbachia* bacteria was made the approach towards LF has been changed. *Wolbachia* in *B. malayi* activates TLR2-TLR6 interactions which in turn triggers the adaptor molecules MyD88 and TIRAP/Mal causing innate inflammatory events (Hise *et al.,* 2004). Purified major Wolbachia surface protein (rWSP) acts as a ligand to TLR2 and TLR4 (Table **3**) [10].

Table 3. Ligands that bind with TLRs from filarial parasites.

Ligand	Pathogen	TLR	Reference
sheath antigen protein	*Wuchereriabancrofti*	**TLR 4**	Mukherjee, *et al.,* 2019 [10]
Lacto-N-fucopentose III	filarial parasite	**TLR 4**	Goodridge, *et al.,* 2005) [10]
phosphorylcholine-decoratedglycans	filarial parasite	**TLR 4**	Goodridge, *et al.,* 2005) [10]
Brugiapahangi antigen (BpA)	*Brugiapahangi*	**TLR4**	(Alok Das Mohapatra, *et al.,* 2014). [10]

(Table 3) cont.....

Ligand	Pathogen	TLR	Reference
purified major Wolbachia surface protein (rWSP)	endosymbionts of the genus Wolbachia (Rickettsiales) of filarial nematodes	TLR2 and TLR4	Norbert W. Brattig *et al.*, 2004[10]

Lymphatic Filariasis and Inflammation

In PBMCs of patients with lymphatic pathology, it was shown that vascular endothelial growth factor and angiopoietin levels were increased. Lymphangiogenesis is a process by which new blood vessels form and aggravate the disease. TLRs in lymphatic pathology tend to increase this process and contribute to the pathology [11]. TLR2 and TLR4 are involved in the pathogenesis created by a major surface protein of wolbachia species [12]. Human embryonic skin cells expressing the TLRs are stimulated by *Brugia malayi*. In C57BL/6 and TLR4(-/-) mice filarial extract leads to the production of cytokine production but not from TLR2(-/-) or TLR6(-/-) mice [13]. Murine peritoneal-elicited macrophages were exposed to *Brugia malayi* female worms (bmfe), associated with down-regulation of TLR4 but upregulation of cd14, cd40, and TLR2. But in a TLR2 and MyD88-dependent manner macrophage tolerance is established creating an immunological phenotype that is responsible for human filariasis [14]. In individuals with chronic lymphatic pathology, TLRs have increased production of TH1 in patients with chronic lymphatic pathology. TLR2 and TLR9 are shown to mediate this kind of proinflammatory cytokine production in lymphatic filariasis [15]. In B cells and monocytes of filarial-infected individuals, TLRs expression was lower in the B cells but not in monocytes [16]. Filarial coinfection with latent TB has been shown to diminish the expression of antigen-specific TLR2 and 9 levels in human patients [17]. Mf-Exposed Monocyte-Derived Human Dcs (Mhdcs) Upon Infection With filarial in humans, has shown diminished expression of TLR3 and TLR4 mRNA levels along with the downregulation of various interferons and interleukins [18]. TLR2 And TLR6 are involved in the *Brugia malayi* female extract-induced inflammation [19]. TLR 2 -196 to -173 del polymorphisms is also found to be involved in the bancroftian filariasis in western tanzania.In filarial-infected individuals, TLR expression is monitored in B cells and monocytes in comparison with uninfected individuals and it was found that B cells are having less TLR expression [20]. Dendritic cells also tend to express lesser TLR 3 and 4 upon infection with live filarial parasites . This may be due to the novel protection mechanisms in the development of filarial pathology .

CONCLUDING REMARKS

Genetic polymorphism also plays an important role in a person enhancing or reducing infections. W.bancrofti infection exerts more symptoms in people who are with single nucleotide polymorphism (SNPs) in TLRs. Thus screening patients with SNPs for *W.bancrofi* and providing awareness to them on the precautions to be taken will help in combating the disease.

CONSENT FOR PUBLICATION

Not applicable.

CONFLICT OF INTEREST

The author declares no conflict of interest, financial or otherwise.

ACKNOWLEDGEMENT

Declared none.

REFERENCES

[1] Nutman TB, Kumaraswami V. Regulation of the immune response in lymphatic filariasis: Perspectives on acute and chronic infection with *Wuchereria bancrofti* in South India. Parasite Immunol 2001; 23(7): 389-99.
[http://dx.doi.org/10.1046/j.1365-3024.2001.00399.x] [PMID: 11472558]

[2] Mukherjee S, Karnam A, Das M, Babu SPS, Bayry J. *Wuchereria bancrofti* filaria activates human dendritic cells and polarizes T helper 1 and regulatory T cells *via* toll-like receptor 4. Commun Biol 2019; 2(1): 169.
[http://dx.doi.org/10.1038/s42003-019-0392-8] [PMID: 31098402]

[3] Mshana HJ, Ngowi SX, Baraka V. Role of toll-like receptor 2 (TLR 2). Genetic Polymorphisms in Modulating Susceptibility to Clinical Disease in Wuchereria Bancrofti 2020; 2: 1-5.

[4] Hübner MP, Thomas Stocker J, Mitre E. Inhibition of type 1 diabetes in filaria-infected non-obese diabetic mice is associated with a T helper type 2 shift and induction of FoxP3 + regulatory T cells. Immunology 2009; 127(4): 512-22.
[http://dx.doi.org/10.1111/j.1365-2567.2008.02958.x] [PMID: 19016910]

[5] Taylor MJ, Cross HF, Bilo K. Inflammatory responses induced by the filarial nematode *Brugia malayi* are mediated by lipopolysaccharide-like activity from endosymbiotic Wolbachia bacteria. J Exp Med 2000; 191(8): 1429-36.
[http://dx.doi.org/10.1084/jem.191.8.1429] [PMID: 10770808]

[6] Turner JD, Langley RS, Johnston KL, *et al.* Wolbachia lipoprotein stimulates innate and adaptive immunity through Toll-like receptors 2 and 6 to induce disease manifestations of filariasis. J Biol Chem 2009; 284(33): 22364-78.
[http://dx.doi.org/10.1074/jbc.M901528200] [PMID: 19458089]

[7] Babu S, Blauvelt CP, Kumaraswami V, Nutman TB. Diminished expression and function of TLR in lymphatic filariasis: A novel mechanism of immune dysregulation. J Immunol 2005; 175(2): 1170-6.
[http://dx.doi.org/10.4049/jimmunol.175.2.1170] [PMID: 16002719]

[8] Goodridge HS, Marshall FA, Else KJ, *et al.* Immunomodulation *via* novel use of TLR4 by the filarial

nematode phosphorylcholine-containing secreted product, ES-62. J Immunol 2005; 174(1): 284-93. [http://dx.doi.org/10.4049/jimmunol.174.1.284] [PMID: 15611251]

[9] Molteni M, Gemma S, Rossetti C. The role of toll-like receptor 4 in infectious and noninfectious inflammation. Mediators Inflamm 2016; 2016 [http://dx.doi.org/10.1155/2016/6978936]

[11] Babu S, Anuradha R, Kumar NP, George PJ, Kumaraswami V, Nutman TB. Toll-like receptor- and filarial antigen-mediated, mitogen-activated protein kinase- and nf-κb-dependent regulation of angiogenic growth factors in filarial lymphatic pathology. Infect immun 2012; 80(7): 2509-18. [http://dx.doi.org/10.1128/IAI.06179-11]

[12] Brattig NW, Bazzocchi C, Kirschning CJ, *et al.* The major surface protein of Wolbachia endosymbionts in filarial nematodes elicits immune responses through TLR2 and TLR4. J Immunol 2004; 173(1): 437-45. [http://dx.doi.org/10.4049/jimmunol.173.1.437] [PMID: 15210803]

[13] Hise AG, Daehnel K, Gillette-Ferguson I, *et al.* Innate immune responses to endosymbiotic Wolbachia bacteria in *Brugia malayi* and Onchocerca volvulus are dependent on TLR2, TLR6, MyD88, and Mal, but not TLR4, TRIF, or TRAM. J Immunol 2007; 178(2): 1068-76. [http://dx.doi.org/10.4049/jimmunol.178.2.1068] [PMID: 17202370]

[14] Turner JD, Langley RS, Johnston KL, Egerton G, Wanji S, Taylor MJ. Wolbachia endosymbiotic bacteria of *Brugia malayi* mediate macrophage tolerance to TLR- and CD40-specific stimuli in a MyD88/TLR2-dependent manner. J Immunol 2006; 177(2): 1240-9. [http://dx.doi.org/10.4049/jimmunol.177.2.1240] [PMID: 16818783]

[15] Babu S, Anuradha R, Kumar NP, George PJ, Kumaraswami V, Nutman TB. Filarial lymphatic pathology reflects augmented toll-like receptor-mediated, mitogen-activated protein kinase-mediated proinflammatory cytokine production. Infect Immun 2011; 79(11): 4600-8. [http://dx.doi.org/10.1128/IAI.05419-11] [PMID: 21875961]

[16] Babu S, Bhat SQ, Kumar NP, *et al.* Attenuation of toll-like receptor expression and function in latent tuberculosis by coexistent filarial infection with restoration following antifilarial chemotherapy. PLoS Negl Trop Dis 2009; 3(7): e489. [http://dx.doi.org/10.1371/journal.pntd.0000489] [PMID: 19636364]

[17] Semnani RT, Venugopal PG, Leifer CA, Mostböck S, Sabzevari H, Nutman TB. Inhibition of TLR3 and TLR4 function and expression in human dendritic cells by helminth parasites. Blood 2008; 112(4): 1290-8. [http://dx.doi.org/10.1182/blood-2008-04-149856]

[18] Turner JD, Langley RS, Johnston KL, Gentil K. Wolbachia lipoprotein stimulates innate and adaptive immunity through toll-like receptors 2 and 6 to induce disease manifestations of filariasis. J biol chem 2009; 284(33): 22364-78. [http://dx.doi.org/10.1074/jbc.M901528200]

[19] Semnani RT, Venugopal PG, Leifer CA, Mostbock S, Sabzevari H, Nutman TB. Inhibition of TLR3 and TLR4 function and expression in human dendritic cells by helminth parasites. Blood 2008; 112: 1290-8.

[20] Venugopal PG, Nutman TB, Semnani RT. Activation and regulation of toll-like receptors (TLRs) by helminth parasites. Immunol Res 2009; 43: 252-63.

CHAPTER 5

TLRs and Visceral *Leishmania*sis

Abstract: Sandly bites transmit the *Leishmania* parasites under the skin, and the disease remains a major public health problem in infected countries. There are two types of *Leishmania*sis, 1) Visceral *Leishmania*sis 2) cutaneous *Leishmania*sis. Among these two types, Visceral *Leishmania*sis is fatal, and, if not treated, leads to mortality. It is observed that approximately 90% of cases come from India, Bangladesh, Sudan, South Sudan, Ethiopia, and Brazil. These diseases are caused by *L. major*, *L. mexicana, L. guyanensis*, *L. amazonensis*, *L. braziliensis*, and visceral *Leishmania*sis by *L. donovani*, and *L. chagasi*. Experimental studies in KO of TLR2 and TLR4 have shown larger lesions and higher parasite loads upon infection with *L. mexicana* than the control mice [1]. *Leishmania* DNA is recognised as a PAMP by TLR9 [2]. These parasites are rapidly phagocytosized by neutrophils, macrophages, and dendritic cells. Different parasites of *Leishmania* elicit different kinds of responses in the host, which in turn depends on the genetics and immune responses of the host.

Keywords: *L. braziliensis*, *L.chagasi*, *L. donovani*, *L. major*, *L. major*, Pegylated bisacycloxypropylcysteine.

INTRODUCTION

TLR 2 is activated upon cutaneous *Leishmania*sis and cytokine overexpression is also noted during visceral *Leishmania*sis [1, 2]. Purified *L. major* lipophosphoglycan (LPG), is a PAMP to TLR2 that activates NK cells [3]. Immunohistochemical expression of TLRs 2,9, and 4 from skin lesions of 40 patients infected with *Leishmania* (V.) braziliensis and *Leishmania*(L.) amazonensis were investigated.This study points out that both pathogens differed in their ability to induce TLRs expression. For example, *L.* (*V.*) *braziliensis* induced higher expression of TLR2 and TLR4 whereas *L.* (*L.*) *amazonensis* showed a strong correlation with the TLR9 [4], Further studies corroborate that active *Leishmania* cases display increased expression of TLR2 and TLR4 along with other cytokines such as TNF-α, IL-10, and TGF-β [5]. However, after drug treatment, there was a sliding of cells from pro and anti-inflammation even under the expression of TLRs.

Monocyte cell lines infected with *Leishmania* parasites showed downregulation of TLR2 and TLR4, causing an increase in IL-10 and IL-12p40 production [6]. The

Jayalakshmi Krishnan

parasite uses this kind of mechanism for its survival, also the study showed that parasite structural integrity is important for its modulation of pathways *via* TLR2 [7]. However, at the initial stages of infection with *L.chagasi*there is an increase in the TLR2-4, IL-17, TNF-α and TGF-β mRNA expression however at later stages of infection there is a decreased expression leading to immunomodulatory events.

Some natural ligands for TLRs act as a protective mechanism for *Leishmania* infection.

For example, Pegylated Bisacycloxypropylcysteine, a Diacylated Lipopeptide (BPPcysMPEG,) provides anti-*Leishmania*l protection by inducing the IL-12, T regulatory cells and Nitric oxide in BALB/c-derived peritoneal macrophages upon infection with *L. major* [8, 9]. For any therapeutic approaches, this kind of mechanism can further be explored. Progmastigotes and amastigotes differ in their capacity to display Glycocalyx. Amastigotes do not possess the glycocalyx layer, suggesting that promastigotes would preserve this structure, whereas amastigotes lose it during intracellular transformation.

Through adaptor molecule MyD88 of TLRs produce IL-1α in macrophages. These findings came from the studies which were done on MyD88-/- cells (Hawn *et al.,* 2002). T cell, maturation, and DC priming are dependent on MyD88 and TLRs during *Leishmania* infection. *L. donovani*, *L. braziliensis*, *L. major,* and *L. mexicana* were found to induce DC maturation during the presence of MyD88, whereas the absence of MyD88 attenuated these process (De Trez *et al.,* 2004). Two antigens from *L. donovani* (65 and 98 kDa, in combination) in the macrophage cell line have upregulated TLR2 expression (Srivastava *et al.,* 2011). In human primary macrophages, *L. panamensis, infection caused an upregualtion various TLRs such as* TLR1, TLR2, TLR3, and TLR4 along with the secretion of TNF. Both amastigotes and promastigotes of *L. panamensis,* have failed to induce the TNF production in MyD88/TRIF$^{-/-}$ murine bone marrow-derived macrophages and mouse macrophage cell lines [10]. Interestingly, at the early stages of parasite infection, the absence of TNFa in TLR4-/- macrophage cells caused increased parasite survival. TLR2 absence does not alter the production of TNFa to the infection by *L. panamensis,* whereas TLR4, as well as endosomal TLRs, are indispensible for macrophage activation (Table **4**).

Table 4. Visceral *Leishmaniasis*: Ligand and TLRs.

Ligand	TLR	Ref
L. donovani promastigotes	TLR2 and 3	Flandin *et al.*, 2006
LPGs of *L. major*, *L. mexicana*, *L. aethiopica*, and *L. tropica*	TLR2 ligands	de Veer *et al.*, 2003, Srivastava*et al.*, 2013
L. donovani antigens (65 and 98 kDa, in combination)	TLR2	Srivastava *et al.*, 2011 [11]

Mice lacking MyD88, an adaptor protein of TLR pathways, seems to be more susceptible to *L. major* infection than the wild-type C57BL/6 MICE [12]. By TLR2 pathways, the lipophosphoglycan (lpg) i from *L. major* is involved in eliciting the immune response. TLKRs not only recognize protozoan PAMPs but also they can recognize bacterial and fungal ligands as well. TLR2 can be activated upon binding with T.cruzi *via* glycosylphosphatidylinositol (gpi) anchors [13]. Mice lacking TLR2,4, 1 infected with *L. major* have displayed a significant increase in parasitic burden along with large lesions by promoting TH2 immunity [14]. *L. Major* IR75 infection with MyD88 -/- is causing the susceptibility of the mice to the infection due to impaired Th1 responses [15]. TLR9 knockout mice displayed the highest susceptibility to T.cruzi infection due to the IL12/IFN responses in antigen-presenting cells [16]. Anti*Leishmania*l responses are mediated by decreased expression of TLR9 in BLAB/c mice [17]. In susceptible balb/c mice, it was observed that TLR has interdependency on each other for eliciting immune responses upon infection with *Leishmania Major* [18] .

The same observations were made in susceptible balb/c mice have elicited strong anti-Leishmanial function through CD40 along with TLR4 to *Leishmania Major* [19]. Infection of macrophages with *L. major* has resulted in reducing TLR9-induced anti Leishmanial responses by downregulating TLR9 *via* interaction with lipophosphoglycan and TLR2 [20]. C57bl/6 mice defective in TLR3,7 and 9 are tested for their capacity for autophagy in macrophages after Leishmania infection and it was found that the cells undergo autophagy and lead the path to the resistance of the parasite . In C57bl/6 Mice, TLR3,4 And 9 By inducing Interferon Interleukin responses cause resistance to the *L. Major* infection [21]. *L. major* promastigotes infection in TLR9 deficient macrophages display decreased expression of TLR1,2 and 3 also these macrophages display less CD40 and interleukin 12 expressions [22]. In macrophages treated with *L. major* infection has reduced CD 40 expression which in turn leads to reduced infection through the N-RAS activation [23]. *Leishmania major*-infected macrophages cause interleukin-dependent T regulatory cells induced anti-Leishmanial protection for pegylated bisacycloxypropylcysteine a TLR6 ligand . In mouse peritoneal macrophages, activation of TLR7 with imidazoquinolines lead to the production of free radicals and cytokines against *L. amazonensis* [24]. From Cutaneous *Leishmaniasis* In Humans the monocytes have produced TLR2/4 expression followed by TNF production infected with *Leishmania braziliensis* [25]. Blockdade of TLR in *Leishmania braziliensis* infection from human cutaneous *Leishmaniasis* has reduced host immune responses [26]. American tegumentary *Leishmaniasis* (atl) is caused by *Leishmania braziliensis*. By PCR reaction the human patients with this disease were evaluated and found that macrophages express more TLR2 in response to the infection [27]. In VL patients TLR2 and TLR4 were involved in the modulation of cytokine production after the treatment of drugs. However, there were lower TNF alpha and nitric oxide levels . In the acute and chronic phases of infection, there was a modulation of TLR-dependent cytokines in mice upon infection with *Leishmania chagasi* [32]. TLR4 gene polymorphisms at 896 and 1196 are not a major factor in contributing to the in patients from Iran infected with visceral *Leishmaniasis* [28]. In the acute and chronic phases of infection, there was a modulation of TLR- dependent cytokines in mice upon infection with *Leishmania chagasi* [29].

Mice infected with *L. chagasi* have differential expression of various cytokines and TLRs expression in the spleen cells [29]. In c57bl/6 mice, *Leishmania donovani* infection has caused upregulation of TLR4 and downregulation of TLR2 [30]. TLR4(-/-) mice upon infection have shown fewer interferons, TNF, and iNOS synthesis [31]. *Leishmania donovani* Infection Targets TLR 2,3, And 4 and abolished IFN-B Gene Expression In *TLR2*$^{-/-}$ Macrophages [31]. *L. major* infection in raw cells protein kinase c mediates the death of the parasite by TLR activation followed by TNF [32]. People infected with visceral *Leishmaniasis* from sudan showed higher TLR9 and TLR4 in their blood samples. THP human cell line upon infection upregulated IL-10 production upon infection with *L. donovani* promastigotes. Interefron gamma primed macrophages have given the *L. donovani* promastigotes as infection and was shown that they upregulate the TLR4 expression after the priming. Genotypes are also found to be the reason for *Leishmaniasis* infection [33].

For example, TLR4 asp299gly and thr399ile genotypes are reported to be the main reason for visceral *Leishmania*sis in Indian patients [34]. Diffuse Cutaneous *Leishmania*sis (Dcl) is shown to produce reduced TLR2, TLR1, And TLR6 in comparison with localised cutaneous *Leishmania*sis, followed by reduced NK cell responses thus causing the disease more severe [35]. In cutaneous *Leishmania*sis patients, macrophages express higher TLR2 in the healing form of the disease than in patients with a non healing form of the disease [36]. *L. tropica* exposed macrophages express TLR2-9 and TNF in comparison with an unexposed group [43]. The synergistic action of TLR with NK cells also contributes to the immunotherapy of *Leishmania*sis by eliciting interferon responses [37]. TLR2 plays an important role in specific and strain-specific induction of inflammatory responses to various *Leishmania* pathogens [38]. To elicit the anti-*Leishmania*l functions TLR2 dimerization along with PKC isoforms works in the targeted therapy [39]. In BALB/C mice with L.donovani infection, it was noted T cell-dependent responses are mediated by colocalization on dectin 1 and TLR2. In macrophages, this ligation elicits strong signaling through Myd88 pathways [40]. In spleen tissue, there was a high expression of TLR 2 and 4 upon infection with visceral *Leishmania*sis with an absent expression of TLR9 [41]. In mice, myledoid dendritic cells require the expression of TLR9 upon *Leishmania*l infection for NK cell activation for IFN gamma release [42]. *L. major* -infected macrophages treated with nanocapsule antigen of TLR agonists cause protection from the parasite [43]. There are differences in protective and non-protective immune responses in the infection caused by various *Leishmania* parasites [44]. For example, *L. infantum* and *L. Mexicana* trigger the TLR2/9 causing protective immune responses whereas *L. major* and *L. amazonensis* cause the TLR2/9 related responses which are not protective [45]. Silencing of TLR11/12 increased interferon-gamma production but reduces the parasite burden in macrophages further reducing the interleukin levels [46].

CONCLUDING REMARKS

During clinical manifestations it's seen that there is a compromise in the host immune responses, leading to a failure in innate immune responses. This also accompanies decreased Th1 cell response, decreased macrophage activation, and increased Th2 production may be due to the inactive nature of TLRs. *Leishmania* has various antigens and the developmental stages of the parasite may vary but stimulate the immune system.

CONSENT FOR PUBLICATION

Not applicable.

CONFLICT OF INTEREST

The author declares no conflict of interest, financial or otherwise.

ACKNOWLEDGEMENT

Declared none.

REFERENCES

[1] Halliday A, Bates PA, Chance ML, Taylor MJ. Toll-like receptor 2 (TLR2) plays a role in controlling cutaneous *Leishmania*sis *in vivo*, but does not require activation by parasite lipophosphoglycan. Parasit

Vectors 2016; 9(1): 532.
[http://dx.doi.org/10.1186/s13071-016-1807-8] [PMID: 27716391]

[2] Babiker DT, Bakhiet SM, Mukhtar MM. *Leishmania* donovani influenced cytokines and Toll-like receptors expression among Sudanese visceral *Leishmania*sis patients. Parasite Immunol 2015; 37(8): 417-25.
[http://dx.doi.org/10.1111/pim.12202] [PMID: 25982946]

[3] Becker I, Salaiza N, Aguirre M, *et al. Leishmania* lipophosphoglycan (LPG) activates NK cells through toll-like receptor-2. Mol Biochem Parasitol 2003; 130(2): 65-74.
[http://dx.doi.org/10.1016/S0166-6851(03)00160-9] [PMID: 12946842]

[4] Campos MB, Lima LVR, de Lima ACS, *et al.* Toll-like receptors 2, 4, and 9 expressions over the entire clinical and immunopathological spectrum of American cutaneous *Leishmania*sis due to *Leishmania* (V.) braziliensis and *Leishmania* (L.) amazonensis. PLoS One 2018; 13(3)e0194383
[http://dx.doi.org/10.1371/journal.pone.0194383] [PMID: 29543867]

[5] Gatto M, de Abreu MM, Tasca KI, *et al.* The involvement of TLR2 and TLR4 in cytokine and nitric oxide production in visceral *Leishmania*sis patients before and after treatment with anti-*Leishmania*l drugs. PLoS One 2015; 10(2)e0117977
[http://dx.doi.org/10.1371/journal.pone.0117977] [PMID: 25706930]

[6] Chandra D, Naik S. *Leishmania* donovani infection down-regulates TLR2-stimulated IL-12p40 and activates IL-10 in cells of macrophage/monocytic lineage by modulating MAPK pathways through a contact-dependent mechanism. Clin Exp Immunol 2008; 154(2): 224-34.
[http://dx.doi.org/10.1111/j.1365-2249.2008.03741.x] [PMID: 18778366]

[7] Srivastava S, Pandey SP, Jha MK, Chandel HS, Saha B. *Leishmania* expressed lipophosphoglycan interacts with Toll-like receptor (TLR)-2 to decrease TLR-9 expression and reduce anti-*Leishmania*l responses. Clin Exp Immunol 2013; 172(3): 403-9.
[http://dx.doi.org/10.1111/cei.12074] [PMID: 23600828]

[8] Pandey SP, Chandel HS, Srivastava S, *et al.* Pegylated bisacycloxypropylcysteine, a diacylated lipopeptide ligand of TLR6, plays a host-protective role against experimental *Leishmania major* infection. J Immunol 2014; 193(7): 3632-43.
[http://dx.doi.org/10.4049/jimmunol.1400672] [PMID: 25194056]

[9] Pimenta PFP, Saraiva EMB, Sacks DL. The comparative fine structure and surface glycoconjugate expression of three life stages of *Leishmania major*. Exp Parasitol 1991; 72(2): 191-204.
[http://dx.doi.org/10.1016/0014-4894(91)90137-L] [PMID: 2009923]

[10] Gallego C, Golenbock D, Gomez MA, Saravia NG. Toll-like receptors participate in macrophage activation and intracellular control of *Leishmania* (Viannia) *panamensis*. Infect Immun 2011; 79(7): 2871-9.
[http://dx.doi.org/10.1128/IAI.01388-10] [PMID: 21518783]

[11] Srivastava A, Singh N, Mishra M, *et al.* Identification of TLR inducing Th1-responsive *Leishmania donovani* amastigote-specific antigens. Mol Cell Biochem 2012; 359(1-2): 359-68.
[http://dx.doi.org/10.1007/s11010-011-1029-5] [PMID: 21858498]

[12] de Veer MJ, Curtis JM, Baldwin TM, *et al.* MyD88 is essential for clearance of *Leishmania major*: possible role for lipophosphoglycan and Toll-like receptor 2 signaling. Eur J Immunol 2003; 33(10): 2822-31.
[http://dx.doi.org/10.1002/eji.200324128] [PMID: 14515266]

[13] Campos MA, Almeida IC, Takeuchi O, *et al.* Activation of toll-like receptor-2 by glycosylphosphatidylinositol anchors from a protozoan parasite. j. immuno 2001; 167: 416-23.

[14] Halliday A, Bates PA, Chance ML, Taylor MJ. Toll-like receptor 2 (TLR2) plays a role in controlling cutaneous *Leishmania*sis *in vivo*, but does not require activation by parasite lipophosphoglycan. Parasit Vectors 2016; 9(1): 532.
[http://dx.doi.org/10.1186/s13071-016-1807-8] [PMID: 27716391]

[15] Revaz-Breton M, Ronet C, Ives A, *et al.* The MyD88 protein 88 pathway is differently involved in immune responses induced by distinct substrains of *Leishmania major*. Eur J Immunol 2010; 40(6): 1697-707. [http://dx.doi.org/10.1002/eji.200939821] [PMID: 20333623]

[16] Bafica A, Santiago HC, Goldszmid R, Ropert C, Gazzinelli RT, Sher A. Cutting edge: TLR9 and TLR2 signaling together account for MyD88-dependent control of parasitemia in *Trypanosoma cruzi* infection. J Immunol 2006; 177(6): 3515-9. [http://dx.doi.org/10.4049/jimmunol.177.6.3515] [PMID: 16951309]

[17] PANDEY SP, JHA MK, CHANDEL HS, SAHA B. *Leishmania* expressed lipophosphoglycan interacts with toll-like receptor (TLR)-2 to decrease TLR-9 expression and reduce anti- *Leishmania*l responses. Clin Exp Immunol 2013; 172(403)

[18] Shukla D, Patidar A, Sarma U, *et al.* Interdependencies between Toll-like receptors in *Leishmania* infection. Immunology 2021; 164(1): 173-89. [http://dx.doi.org/10.1111/imm.13364] [PMID: 33964011]

[19] Chandel HS, Pandey SP, Shukla D, *et al.* Toll-like receptors and CD40 modulate each other's expression affecting *Leishmania* major infection. Clin Exp Immunol 2014; 176(2): 283-90. [http://dx.doi.org/10.1111/cei.12264] [PMID: 24387292]

[20] Franco LH, Fleuri AKA, Pellison NC, *et al.* Autophagy downstream of endosomal Toll-like receptor signaling in macrophages is a key mechanism for resistance to *Leishmania* major infection. J Biol Chem 2017; 292(32): 13087-96. [http://dx.doi.org/10.1074/jbc.M117.780981] [PMID: 28607148]

[21] Schamber-Reis BLF, Petritus PM, Caetano BC, *et al.* UNC93B1 and nucleic acid-sensing Toll-like receptors mediate host resistance to infection with *Leishmania major*. J Biol Chem 2013; 288(10): 7127-36. [http://dx.doi.org/10.1074/jbc.M112.407684] [PMID: 23325805]

[22] Pandey SP, Doyen N, Mishra GC, Saha B, Chandel HS. TLR9-deficiency reduces TLR1, TLR2 and TLR3 expressions in *Leishmania* major-infected macrophages. Exp Parasitol 2015; 154: 82-6. [http://dx.doi.org/10.1016/j.exppara.2015.04.005] [PMID: 25911242]

[23] Chakraborty S, Srivastava A, Jha MK, *et al.* Inhibition of CD40-induced N-Ras activation reduces *Leishmania major* infection. J Immunol 2015; 194(8): 3852-60. [http://dx.doi.org/10.4049/jimmunol.1401996] [PMID: 25786685]

[24] Kaushik D, Granato JT, Macedo GC, *et al.* Toll-like receptor-7/8 agonist kill *Leishmania* amazonensis by acting as pro-oxidant and pro-inflammatory agent. J Pharm Pharmacol 2021; 73(9): 1180-90. [http://dx.doi.org/10.1093/jpp/rgab063] [PMID: 33940589]

[25] Polari LP, Carneiro PP, Macedo M, *et al.* *Leishmania* braziliensis infection enhances toll-like receptors 2 and 4 expression and triggers Tnf-α and IL-10 production in human cutaneous *Leishmania*sis. Front Cell Infect Microbiol 2019; 9: 120. [http://dx.doi.org/10.3389/fcimb.2019.00120] [PMID: 31119102]

[26] Carneiro PP, Dórea AS, Oliveira WN, *et al.* blockade of TLR2 and TLR4 attenuates inflammatory response and parasite load in cutaneous *Leishmania*sis. Front Immunol 2021; 12706510 [http://dx.doi.org/10.3389/fimmu.2021.706510] [PMID: 34691019]

[27] Tuon FF, Fernandes ER, Duarte MIS, Amato VS. Expression of TLR2 and TLR4 in lesions of patients with tegumentary american *Leishmania*sis. Rev Inst Med Trop São Paulo 2012; 54(3): 159-64. [http://dx.doi.org/10.1590/S0036-46652012000300008] [PMID: 22634888]

[28] Rasouli M, Keshavarz M, Kalani M, *et al.* toll-like receptor 4 (TLR4) polymorphisms in iranian patients with visceral leishmaniasis. mol biol rep 39, 2012; 10795-802.

[29] Cezário GAG, Oliveira LRC, Peresi E, *et al.* Analysis of the expression of toll-like receptors 2 and 4 and cytokine production during experimental *Leishmania* chagasi infection. Mem Inst Oswaldo Cruz

2011; 106(5): 573-83.
[http://dx.doi.org/10.1590/S0074-02762011000500010] [PMID: 21894379]

[30] Murray HW, Zhang Y, Zhang Y, Raman VS, Reed SG, Ma X. Regulatory actions of toll-like receptor 2 (TLR2) and TLR4 in leishmania donovani infection in the liver. infect immun. 2013; 81(7): 2318-6.

[31] Dias BT, Goundry A, Vivarini AC, *et al.* Toll-like receptor- and protein kinase r-induced type I interferon sustains infection of *Leishmania* donovani in macrophages. Front Immunol 2022; 13801182
[http://dx.doi.org/10.3389/fimmu.2022.801182] [PMID: 35154115]

[32] Faria MS, Calegari-Silva TC, Vivarini AC, Mottram JC, Lopes UG, Lima APCA. Role of protein kinase R in the killing of *Leishmania* major by macrophages in response to neutrophil elastase and TLR4 *via* TNFα and IFNβ. FASEB J 2014; 28(7): 3050-63.
[http://dx.doi.org/10.1096/fj.13-245126] [PMID: 24732131]

[33] Flandin JF, Chano F, Descoteaux A. RNA interference reveals a role for TLR2 and TLR3 in the recognition *of Leishmania donovani* promastigotes by interferon–γ-primed macrophages. Eur J Immunol 2006; 36(2): 411-20.
[http://dx.doi.org/10.1002/eji.200535079] [PMID: 16369915]

[34] Mandal A, Kumar M, Kumar A, Sen A, Das P, Das S. TLR4 and TLR9 polymorphism: probable role in susceptibility among the population of bihar for indian visceral leishmaniasis. innate immun. 2021; 27(6): 493-500.

[35] Cañeda-Guzmán IC, Salaiza-Suazo N, Fernández-Figueroa EA, Carrada-Figueroa G, Aguirre-García M, Becker I. NK cell activity differs between patients with localized and diffuse cutaneous *Leishmania*sis infected with *Leishmania mexicana* : a comparative study of TLRs and cytokines. PLoS One 2014; 9(11)e112410
[http://dx.doi.org/10.1371/journal.pone.0112410] [PMID: 25397678]

[36] Tolouei S, Hejazi SH, Ghaedi K, Khamesipour A, Hasheminia SJ. TLR2 and TLR4 in cutaneous *Leishmania*sis caused by *Leishmania major* . Scand J Immunol 2013; 78(5): 478-84.
[http://dx.doi.org/10.1111/sji.12105] [PMID: 23980810]

[37] Oliaee RT, Sharifi I, Afgar A, *et al.* Differential expression of TLRs 2, 4, 9, iNOS and TNF-α and arginase activity in peripheral blood monocytes from glucantime unresponsive and responsive patients with anthroponotic cutaneous *Leishmania*sis caused by *Leishmania* tropica. Microb Pathog 2019; 126: 368-78.
[http://dx.doi.org/10.1016/j.micpath.2018.11.004] [PMID: 30399441]

[38] Karmakar S, Bhaumik SK, Paul J, De T. TLR4 and NKT cell synergy in immunotherapy against visceral *Leishmania*sis. PLoS Pathog 2012; 8(4)e1002646
[http://dx.doi.org/10.1371/journal.ppat.1002646] [PMID: 22511870]

[39] Mukherjee A, Roy S, Patidar A, *et al.* TLR2 dimer-specific ligands selectively activate protein kinase c isoforms in Leishmania infection 2021; 164(2): 318-331.
[http://dx.doi.org/10.1111/imm.13373]

[40] Patidar A, Mahanty T, Raybarman C, *et al.* Barley beta-Glucan and Zymosan induce Dectin-1 and Toll-like receptor 2 co-localization and anti-*Leishmania*l immune response in *Leishmania* donovani - infected BALB/c mice. Scand J Immunol 2020; 92(6)e12952
[http://dx.doi.org/10.1111/sji.12952] [PMID: 32748397.]

[41] Kumar R, Singh OP, Gautam S, Nylen S, Sundar S. nhanced expression of toll-like receptors 2 and 4, but not 9, in spleen tissue from patients with visceral leishmaniasis. parasite immunol. 2014; 36(12): 721-5.

[42] Schleicher U, Liese J, Knippertz I, *et al.* NK cell activation in visceral *Leishmania*sis requires TLR9, myeloid DCs, and IL-12, but is independent of plasmacytoid DCs. J Exp Med 2007; 204(4): 893-906.
[http://dx.doi.org/10.1084/jem.20061293] [PMID: 17389237]

[43] Katebi A, Varshochian R, Riazi-rad F, Ganjalikhani-hakemi M, Ajdary S. combinatorial delivery of

antigen and TLR agonists *via* plga nanoparticles modulates leishmania major-infected-macrophages activation. biomed pharmacother 2021; 137: 111276.

[44] Bamigbola IE, Ali S. Paradoxical immune response in *Leishmania*sis: The role of toll-like receptors in disease progression. Parasite Immunol 2022; 44(4-5)e12910 [http://dx.doi.org/10.1111/pim.12910] [PMID: 35119120]

[45] Shukla D, Chandel HS, Srivastava S, *et al.* TLR11 or TLR12 silencing reduces *Leishmania major* infection. Cytokine 2018; 104: 110-3. [http://dx.doi.org/10.1016/j.cyto.2017.10.005] [PMID: 29017773]

[46] Shukla D, Chandel HS, Srivastava S, *et al.* TLR11 or TLR12 silencing reduces *Leishmania major* infection. Cytokine 2018; 104: 110-3. [http://dx.doi.org/10.1016/j.cyto.2017.10.005] [PMID: 29017773]

CHAPTER 6

Dengue Virus and Toll-Like Receptors

Abstract: Dengue is one of the most important arboviral diseases recorded in the world. Dengue, a public health problem in tropical and subtropical countries, is spread by female *Aedes* mosquito bites. Among *Aedes* mosquitoes, *Aedesaegypti* is the primary vector and *Aedesalbopictus* is the less infective secondary vector [1]. Dengue hemorrhagic fever (DHF) is a severe form of the disease, that causes differential expression of the TLRs in dendritic cells (DCs). TLR3 and TLR9 in DCs of patients with early onset of dengue fever were unregulated, whereas in severe cases, poor expression of TLR3 and TLR9 is observed [2]. This kind of alteration in the TLR expression during dengue may alter the clinical manifestation of the disease. However, this can be considered for further research on therapeutics.

Keywords: Human peripheral blood mononuclear cells (PBMC), NF-kB mediated pathways.

INTRODUCTION

In blood monocytes, the TLR2 is able to sense the dengue virus infection and modulate the immune responses. TLR2 inhibition to block before dengue infection resulted in the inhibition of NF-kB protein in paediatric patients. Similar studies on severe cases of dengue and other febrile illness have shown differential expression of TLRs.

In cultured hepatoma cells, induction of IFN beta abrogates the type II dengue virus infection which is mediated or activated by TLR3 [3]. This kind of protection mediated by TLR3, can be further explored for therapeutic and clinical prevention of the disease[3]. In the Human peripheral blood mononuclear cells (PBMC), dengue NS1 protein-induced IL6 and TNF production *via* the activation of TLR2 and TLR6. Further, animal studies on TLR6$^{-/-}$ mice treated with DV NS1 protein, have shown higher survivability [4].

The interaction between the virus and the receptor is very complex. Dengue virus infection leads to plasma leakage and increased vascular permeability. There are several groups trying to understand these mechanisms. One such mechanism of immunomodulatory action of the TLR 2 receptor seems to be through the abrogation of NF-kB mediated pathways during TLR2 blockage in blood mono-

Jayalakshmi Krishnan

cytes [5]. Blocking TLR2 prior to DNEV infection prevents the vascular damage caused by the virus by reducing or completely preventing the activation of vascular endothelium.

During NS1 protein stimulation Endocan mRNA levels were higher in the endothelial cell lines [6]. However, the blockade of TLR4 prevented Endocan production in endothelial cells during NS1 activation. Endothelial cell monolayer integrity is disrupted by NS1 (dengue virus non-structural protein) which acts as PMAP by a TLR4-dependent mechanism [7]. This NS1 also acts like LPS-induced inflammatory patterns which are a TLR4 agonist. NS1 protein may induce chemokines and cytokines leading to a vascular leak in dengue-affected patients, thus TLR4 antagonists can offer a therapeutic option.

Almost all human cells express TLRs, especially TLR3, 7, and 9 are seen in various cells of the body such as neurons, epithelial cells, dendritic cells (DCS), lining the airway, genital tract, biliary tract, and intestine. TLRs are always vulnerable to SNPs and these SPNs contribute to the manifestation of various viral and non-viral diseases [8 - 11].

TLR9 (rs187084, rs5743836) and TLR7 (rs179008, rs179009) SNPs are significantly related to the dengue disease in comparison to non-febrile patients. Clinical cases of dengue in Veracruz, Mexico display genetic polymorphism in TLR3, TLR4, TLR7, and TLR8 [12]. The production of IL-6 and TNF-α induced by Dengue virus NS1 protein was found to be reduced when TLR2 and TLR6 receptors were blocked in human PBMC [4]. The same studies extend to animal models such as mice, has also shown the same results. In comparison with Wild type mice infected with Dengue virus NS1 protein, DV NS1 protein-treated TLR6-/- mice have displayed a higher survival rate. NS1 was also found to disrupt the endothelial cell monolayer integrity in *in vitro* model of the vascular leak by activating TLR4 in PBMcs.

Mouse models also suggest that TLR4 antagonists can reduce capillary leak [13, 14]. In comparison with DHF lower expression of LTR2 was found in DF patients. Reduced stimulation of TLR2, TLR9, and no alterations was noticed in TLR4 levels in the Monocytes of patients with severe dengue fever [15]. DENV-antibody complex infection FcR region has downregulated TLRs gene expression and upregulated various other molecules leading to increased viral load [13, 14].

As per a study conducted in human monocytic cells U937 cells, it is shown that IL-8 is secreted after dengue viral detection by TLR3 [16]. Upon the entry of the dengue virus inside the cell, not only TLRs like TLR3 and TLR7, but there are other receptors that sense the dengue virus . These two TLRs are present in endosomes. The other receptors which sense the dengue virus are cytoplasmic retinoic acid-inducible gene I (RIG-I) and melanoma differentiation-associated protein 5 (MDA5). RIG-I, MDA5, and TLR3 combination is crucial in limiting the dengue viral replication and host defense [16].

The knockout studies conducted in HUH-7 cells (silencing RIG-I and MDA5) have led to the high susceptibility of the cell to the virus. Similar observations were made in the same cells when TLR3 is knocked out, leading to high susceptibility. On the other hand, when these cells were silenced only for RIG-I and MDA5, high production of IFN-β was observed. Few other studies confirm the cooperation of RIG-I, MDA5, and TLR3 combination in eliciting strong antiviral responses [17]. In mouse ovarian granulosa cells stimulated with Polyinosinic-polycytidylic acid [poly(I:C)], a TLR3 agonist, lead to the upregulation of TNF-α and IL-6, and type I interferons (IFN-α/β) which are proinflammatory cytokines.TLR3 knockout studies in these cells compromised the production of antiviral responses, also complete abrogation of antiviral response was seen in MDA5/RIG-I signal blocking.

Viral recognition by TLRs triggers a cascade of signalling events such as myeloid differentiation primary response gene 88 (MyD88) and TIR-domain-containing adapter-inducing IFNβ (TRIF) pathways. The result of this pathway activation is to produce pro-inflammatory cytokines such as IFNs. This production of IFNs occurs through the activation of IRF3/IRF7 and nuclear factor-κB (NF-κB). TLR3 and TLR4 are different in sensing ssRNA and dsRNA components. For example, TLR3 binds with dsRNA components and TLR7 binds with ssRNA components. TLR7 activates the myeloid differentiation primary response gene 88-dependent signal pathway whereas TLR3 acts through the TIR-domain-containing adapter-inducing IFNβ. However, the non-structural protein recognition by TLR4 can induce severe vascular damage. Interestingly, dengue virus-infected cells can recognize the viral components through microRNAs [18]. These microRNAs can also be recognized by TLRs, in turn activating innate immune responses. Anti-dengue status can be established in cells through the production of type I IFNs, which are mediated by TLR signaling *via* the activation of transcription factors such as IRF-3, IRF -7 and NF-κB [4, 19].

CONCLUDING REMARKS

Cytokine production is the hallmark of any viral disease and dengue fever is not an exception. Endocan, is a biomarker for endothelial cell activation which result in lymphopenia, and thrombocytopenia results in disease progression. TLR SNPs are reported in various types of diseases such as malaria, TB, lymphatic filariasis, HCV, and cancer.

CONSENT FOR PUBLICATION

Not applicable.

CONFLICT OF INTEREST

The author declares no conflict of interest, financial or otherwise.

ACKNOWLEDGEMENT

Declared none.

REFERENCES

[1] Babiker DT, Bakhiet SM, Mukhtar MM. *Leishmania donovani* influenced cytokines and Toll-like receptors expression among Sudanese visceral leishmaniasis patients. Parasite Immunol 2015; 37(8): 417-25.
[http://dx.doi.org/10.1111/pim.12202] [PMID: 25982946]

[2] Liang Z, Wu S, Li Y, *et al.* Activation of Toll-like receptor 3 impairs the dengue virus serotype 2 replication through induction of IFN-β in cultured hepatoma cells. PLoS One 2011; 6(8): e23346.
[http://dx.doi.org/10.1371/journal.pone.0023346] [PMID: 21829730]

[4] Chen HW, King K, Tu J, Sanchez M, Luster AD, Shresta S. The roles of IRF-3 and IRF-7 in innate antiviral immunity against dengue virus. J Immunol 2013; 191(8): 4194-201.
[http://dx.doi.org/10.4049/jimmunol.1300799] [PMID: 24043884]

[5] Aguilar-Briseño JA, Upasani V, Ellen BM, *et al.* TLR2 on blood monocytes senses dengue virus infection and its expression correlates with disease pathogenesis. Nat Commun 2020; 11(1): 3177.
[http://dx.doi.org/10.1038/s41467-020-16849-7] [PMID: 32576819]

[6] Domínguez-Alemán CA, Sánchez-Vargas LA, Hernández-Flores KG, *et al.* Dengue virus induces the expression and release of endocan from endothelial cells by an ns1–TLR4-dependent mechanism. Microorganisms 2021; 9(6): 1305.
[http://dx.doi.org/10.3390/microorganisms9061305] [PMID: 34203931]

[7] Chao CH, Wu WC, Lai YC, *et al.* Dengue virus nonstructural protein 1 activates platelets *via* Toll-like receptor 4, leading to thrombocytopenia and hemorrhage. PLoS Pathog 2019; 15(4): e1007625.
[http://dx.doi.org/10.1371/journal.ppat.1007625] [PMID: 31009511]

[8] Brown RA, Razonable RR. A real-time PCR assay for the simultaneous detection of functional N284I and L412F polymorphisms in the human Toll-like receptor 3 gene. J Mol Diagn 2010; 12(4): 493-7.
[http://dx.doi.org/10.2353/jmoldx.2010.090122] [PMID: 20413676]

[9] Beima-Sofie K, Wamalwa D, Maleche-Obimbo E, *et al.* Toll-like receptor 9 polymorphism is associated with increased Epstein–Barr virus and Cytomegalovirus acquisition in HIV-exposed infants. AIDS 2018; 32(2): 267-70.
[http://dx.doi.org/10.1097/QAD.0000000000001680] [PMID: 29112074]

[10] Zayed RA, Omran D, Mokhtar DA, *et al.* Association of toll-like receptor 3 and toll-like receptor 9 single nucleotide polymorphisms with Hepatitis C virus infection and hepatic fibrosis in Egyptian patients. Am J Trop Med Hyg 2017; 96(3): 16-0644.
[http://dx.doi.org/10.4269/ajtmh.16-0644] [PMID: 28093541]

[11] Beima-Sofie KM, Bigham AW, Lingappa JR, *et al.* Toll-like receptor variants are associated with infant HIV-1 acquisition and peak plasma HIV-1 RNA level. AIDS 2013; 27(15): 2431-9.
[http://dx.doi.org/10.1097/QAD.0b013e3283629117] [PMID: 24037211]

[12] Posadas-Mondragón A, Aguilar-Faisal JL, Zuñiga G, *et al.* Association of genetic polymorphisms in TLR3, TLR4, TLR7, and TLR8 with the clinical forms of dengue in patients from veracruz, Mexico. Viruses 2020; 12(11): 1230.
[http://dx.doi.org/10.3390/v12111230] [PMID: 33138336]

[13] Modhiran N, Kalayanarooj S, Ubol S. Subversion of innate defenses by the interplay between DENV and pre-existing enhancing antibodies: TLRs signaling collapse. PLoS Negl Trop Dis 2010; 4(12): e924.
[http://dx.doi.org/10.1371/journal.pntd.0000924] [PMID: 21200427]

[14] Modhiran N, Watterson D, Muller DA, *et al.* Dengue virus NS1 protein activates cells *via* Toll-like receptor 4 and disrupts endothelial cell monolayer integrity. Sci Transl Med 2015; 7(304): 304ra142.
[http://dx.doi.org/10.1126/scitranslmed.aaa3863] [PMID: 26355031]

[15] Torres S, Hernández JC, Giraldo D, *et al.* Differential expression of Toll-like receptors in dendritic cells of patients with dengue during early and late acute phases of the disease. PLoS Negl Trop Dis 2013; 7(2): e2060.
[http://dx.doi.org/10.1371/journal.pntd.0002060] [PMID: 23469297]

[16] Nasirudeen AMA, Wong HH, Thien P, Xu S, Lam KP, Liu DX. RIG-I, MDA5 and TLR3 synergistically play an important role in restriction of dengue virus infection. PLoS Negl Trop Dis 2011; 5(1): e926.
[http://dx.doi.org/10.1371/journal.pntd.0000926] [PMID: 21245912]

[17] Yan K, Zhu W, Yu L, *et al.* Toll-like receptor 3 and RIG-I-like receptor activation induces innate antiviral responses in mouse ovarian granulosa cells. Mol Cell Endocrinol 2013; 372(1-2): 73-85.
[http://dx.doi.org/10.1016/j.mce.2013.03.027] [PMID: 23567548]

[18] Urcuqui-Inchima S, Cabrera J, Haenni AL. Interplay between dengue virus and Toll-like receptors, RIG-I/MDA5 and microRNAs: Implications for pathogenesis. Antiviral Res 2017; 147(1): 47-57.
[http://dx.doi.org/10.1016/j.antiviral.2017.09.017] [PMID: 28965915]

[19] Hertzog PJ, O'Neill LA, Hamilton JA. The interferon in TLR signaling: More than just antiviral. Trends Immunol 2003; 24(10): 534-9.
[http://dx.doi.org/10.1016/j.it.2003.08.006] [PMID: 14552837]

CHAPTER 7

Chikungunya Virus and Toll like Receptors

Abstract: Infected mosquitoes of Aedes species spread Chikungunya fever upon the biting of the mosquitoes. Chikungunya fever first came to the limelight upon an outbreak in southern Tanzania in 1952. These days almost all countries in the world are reporting Chikungunya fever. There is no vaccine for the Chikungunya virus. The infection causes severe joint pain, nausea, vomiting, conductivities, headache, and muscle pain, followed by fever. Clinical manifestations occur after 2-7 days of the mosquito bite. This chapter addresses key issues on Chikungunya viral infection in brain cells with reference to the triggering of events associated with toll-like receptors.

Keywords: Chikungunya fever (CHIKF), Chikungunya virus(CHIKV), IFN-α levels, TLR polymorphism in Dengue and CHIKV.

INTRODUCTION

Chikungunya virus_(CHIKV) belongs to the family of *Togaviridae* and the genus of alphaviruses [1]. This virus is transmitted by *Aedes* mosquitoes and the disease caused by the virus became a global public health threat. In 1952 in Tanzania of East Africa first human cases of CHIKV infection have been documented since then there are a lot of countries have reported this virus with endemicity [2]. This virus targets almost all types of cells in the body, such as neuronal cells, dermal cells, fibroblasts, macrophages and monocytes [3 - 5]. Chikungunya fever (CHIKF), is a disease caused by the Chikungunya virus belonging to the family of *Togaviridae*, genus Alphavirus. This is a single-stranded positive virus, upon infection in humans the disease is manifested as myalgia and severe acute or chronic arthralgia [1, 2]. This disease also clinically manifested with immunopathology and the production of alarming levels of pro-inflammatory factors. Among the TLRs, TLR3 seems to contribute or involve in innate immune responses to various viruses such as murine cytomegalovirus, respiratory syncytial virus, influenza virus, Chikungunya virus(CHIKV) and herpes simplex virus 2 [3 - 5].

Type I interferon levels and cytokines are elevated after Chikungunya virus infection as a part of innate immune responses *via* the activation of TLRs. There are studies that explored if genetic variations can be a cause of the development

Jayalakshmi Krishnan

of Chikungunya. One such genetic attribution is due to the presence of the SNPs in genes of TLR8 and TLR7. The presence of SNPs in these receptor genes leads to the patient being more susceptible to Chikungunya [6]. Not only that, possessing the SNPs also renders the cells to make more interferon-alpha. Patients with the rs179010-CC genotype have shown significant production of IFN-α levels [6].

The immunopathological events associated with the CHICK infections seem to be caused by the overproduction of TNFa, and proinflammatory interleukins IL) 1β (IL1β), IL6, IL12p70, and chemokines (CCL2 to CCL 10). The role of TLRs in these immunopathological events is decoded especially through TLRs. It was found that interleukin 27 (IL27) levels were higher in the serum of the patients with chronic chikungunya fever (CHIKF) rather than the acute ones. A study by Valtes-Lopez *et al.,* 2022 has evinced that binding of CHICKV PAMP to TLR1/2-MyD88 activates NF-κB-complex thus leading to EBI3 mRNA which is a heterodimer of IL27. The other pathways during the replicating period of the virus lead to the production of the dsRNA, this binds with TLR3-TRIF leading to the activation of IRF1. This complex in turn leads to the production of IL27 mRNA.

Cytokines and chemokines which are regulated through TLRs have shown differential expression in CSF and serum in patients with and without neurological complications. In patients with neurological complications, in CSF there was an increase in IL-6, IL-8, TNF-α, IFN-α,MCP-1, RANTES, MIG and TARC levels. In patients, without neurological complications, there was a high production of IL-17A, IL-8, IL-1β, MCP-1, RANTES, IP-10 and TARC [7]. This clearly indicates that the TLR system gets activated and sends the inflammatory responses associated with CHIKV infection. In an interesting study by Thangamani *et al.,* 2010 [7], needle-injected CHIKV has upregulated TLR3 transcription and interferon-γ in CD-1 mice, whereas uninfected and mosquito bite has downregulated TLR3 levels. This difference might be due to the composition of the saliva of the mosquito.

There were studies on TLR polymorphism in Dengue and CHIKV co-and mono infections. The study has been done by using eight SNPs of TLR8 (rs5744080-chrX:12919685, rs3764879-chrX:12906578, rs3764880-chrX:12906707) TLR7 (rs179008-chrX:12885540, rs5741880-chrX:12869297, rs179010-chrX:128 84 766, rs3853839-chrX:12889539) and TLR3 (rs3775290-chr4:186083063). In comparison to healthy controls, the co-infected patients display high CC genotypes of TLR8 and 8 SNPs thus rendering the patients to be more susceptible to coinfection [8]. Vitamins are known to establish the antiviral state in a cell, especially a vitamin D3 has been known as an immunomodulator. When the human monocytes (VD3-Mon) and monocyte-derived macrophage cells were infected with CHICKV and Vitamin D3 it has been known to alter the TLR mRNA expression and other proinflammatory cytokines as well. This study highlights the importance of vitamins in the regulation and modulation of innate immunity through TLR signalling [5, 9, 10]. In febrile patients coinfected with Dengue and CHICKV, TLR SNPs are reported to be the CC genotype that causes the susceptible coinfections where as specific genotypes offered protection from both the viral coinfections [11]. In CHICKV-infected macrophages TLR3 induces TRIF a downstream signaling molecule that can cause IRF 1 and TIL27 mRNA expression [12]. Dengue and CHIKCV confection along with various serotypes and especially the dengue 2 serotypes was found to the circulating in the Indian population from west Bengal [13]. Asian lineage CHIKV is reported to suppress DENV replication in infants from mexico [14]. Upon investigation of TLR-induced cytokines in CHICKV patients in serum samples of human patients, it was found that various chemokines and cytokines were without any neuro symptoms. This study proves that TLRs are involved in CHICKV infections [15]. CHICKV susceptibility also increases due to the polymorphisms in TLR-7 and TLR-8 SNPs [16]. Not only that but polymorphisms in TLR3, DC-SIGN, and TNF-α genes were also reported to be involved in the CHICKV infection as reported from the patients from Nicaragua [17]. The same type of study extended to Dengue virus infection is associated with SNPS from rs3775290 for TLR3, followed by SNPS from s8192284 for IL6R, and also rs7248637 for DC-SIGN was reported from the Colombian population [18]. In human and mouse fibroblast cells it was reported that SNPS from TLR on rs6552950 region leads to the severity of the infection [19]. POLY IC an agonist of TLR3 treatment in Human bronchial epithelial cells, inhibited the replication of CHICKV [20]. *TLR7* rs3853839 in male patients causes lymphopenia and increases the risk of infection [21]. TLR polymorphism is reported to be the one form of the manifestations of the disease.

EPIDEMIOLOGY OF CHIKV

CHIKV is reported to be present in the plasma samples of children , and also it was detected in the cerebrospinal fluid of the central nervous system confirming the infection to the nervous system. This was reported from India in 2006 [22]. In La Réunion islands also CHIKV was reported in CSF and plasma the antibodies were found but the antibodies were not seen in the synovial samples and maternal milk [23]. In Salvador, Brazil, out of the many patients admitted due to the fever the screening has resulted in the identification of Zika and CHIKV in at least 20 samples [24]. In the border areas between Colombian and Venezuelan places it was identified that out of the 157 serum samples, the infection of CHIKV was found in 29% of blood samples that is 47 people. This disease was also found to be manifesting with co infections such as ZIKA and Dengue [25]. Same observation was made in Brazil in the year 2015-2016, with a CHIKV genotype of ECSA followed by infections with other arboviruses [26]. In Colombia out of the 23 871 samples tested in the year 2015-2016, it was found that CHIKV-ZIKV coinfection is very common [27].

In Brazil, between 2014 and July 2016 , out of the 948 participants tested, CHIKV has been found in 159 samples followed by other viral diseases such as Dengue and zika virus. Further coinfections with Dengue and CHIKV and *Flavivirus* and CHIKV were also found in many patients [28]. Blood donations were screened for the presence of the dengue (DENV), Chikungunya (CHIKV), and Zika (ZIKV) in Southeast Asia such as Vietnam and Thailand and some samples were tested positive for all three viruses [29]. Even the blood is donated from asymptomatic donors it is necessary to screen it before donating. In the cerebral spinal fluid (CSF) of patients with neurological complications random screening for the virus has revealed the presence of six viral genotypes of CHIKV in western Brazil [30]. In Amapá (AP) and Rio De janiro the co infections with CHIKV and dengue were observed with patients displaying both typical and atypical symptoms [31]. It was the first autochthonous case in Amapa from Brazil and it was then reported in Rio De Janiro as well in 2014 and 2016 respectively. In 2013 in a cross sectional study done at Odisa, India it was seen that out of the 204 samples screened for the presence of dengue and CHIKV, it was reported that 28 patients were identified with CHIKV and 28 people were found to be coinfected with both Dengue and CHIKV. These studies warrant the continuous monitoring of the both the viruses in endemic regions [32]. Similar observations were made in New Delhi in the year 2016, that out of the 130 blood samples tested coinfection of dengue and CHIKV was found in the 9% of blood samples [33]. This study also further reinstates that there should be effective monitoring of the virus in endemic areas. Another study conducted in Delhi in 2016 identified that twenty CHIKV strains were isolated in 87 blood samples by using RT-PCR and IgM ELISA techniques. Similar observations of co infections were made in New Delhi in many patients' blood samples. In Indonesia, it was seen that CHIKV with neurological complications were reported in 4 cases out of 244 cases tested.

CONCLUDING REMARKS

Immunopathological events follow the CHICKV infection leading to the outbreak of cytokines and chemokines. Single nucleotide polymorphisms are also reported to cause the susceptibility of the disease to the virus. RIG I and CHICK virus infections are also linked to each other. Coinfection of the virus with Dengue is also reported to be due to the TLR-mediated signalling cascades.

There are typical and atypical manifestations of the CHIKV fever. The typical manifestations are arthralgia. (pain in knees), myalgia(muscle pain), headaches, exanthema (skin rash) and high fever. Theatypical manifestations include Guillain-Barré syndrome, meningo-encephalitis followed by myeloradiculitis, or combination of both meningoencephalo-myeloradiculitis.

CONSENT FOR PUBLICATION

Not applicable.

CONFLICT OF INTEREST

The author declares no conflict of interest, financial or otherwise.

ACKNOWLEDGEMENT

Declared none.

REFERENCES

[1] Strauss JH, Strauss EG. The alphaviruses: Gene expression, replication, and evolution. Microbiol Rev 1994; 58(3): 491-562.
[http://dx.doi.org/10.1128/mr.58.3.491-562.1994] [PMID: 7968923]

[2] Mason PJ, Haddow AJ. An epidemic of virus disease in Southern Province, Tanganyika Territory, in 1952 53; an additional note on Chikungunya virus isolations and serum antibodies. Trans R Soc Trop Med Hyg 1957; 51(3): 238-40.
[http://dx.doi.org/10.1016/0035-9203(57)90022-6] [PMID: 13443013]

[3] Young AR, Locke MC, Cook LE, *et al.* Dermal and muscle fibroblasts and skeletal myofibers survive chikungunya virus infection and harbor persistent RNA. PLoS Pathog 2019; 15(8): e1007993.
[http://dx.doi.org/10.1371/journal.ppat.1007993] [PMID: 31465513]

[4] Abraham R, McPherson RL, Dasovich M, Badiee M, Leung AKL, Griffin DE. Both ADP-ribosy--binding and hydrolase activities of the alphavirus nsp3 macrodomain affect neurovirulence in mice. MBio 2020; 11(1): e03253-19.
[http://dx.doi.org/10.1128/mBio.03253-19] [PMID: 32047134]

[5] Valdés-López JF, Velilla P, Urcuqui-Inchima S. Vitamin D modulates the expression of Toll-like receptors and pro-inflammatory cytokines without affecting Chikungunya virus replication, in monocytes and macrophages. Acta Trop 2022; 232(1): 106497.
[http://dx.doi.org/10.1016/j.actatropica.2022.106497] [PMID: 35508271]

[6] Valdés-López JF, Fernandez GJ, Urcuqui-Inchima S. Synergistic effects of toll-like receptor 1/2 and toll-like receptor 3 signaling triggering interleukin 27 gene expression in chikungunya virus-infected macrophages. Front Cell Dev Biol 2022; 10(1): 812110.
[http://dx.doi.org/10.3389/fcell.2022.812110] [PMID: 35223841]

[7] Felipe VLJ, Paula A V, Silvio UI. Chikungunya virus infection induces differential inflammatory and antiviral responses in human monocytes and monocyte-derived macrophages. Acta Trop 2020; 211(1): 105619.
[http://dx.doi.org/10.1016/j.actatropica.2020.105619] [PMID: 32634389]

[8] Sengupta S, Mukherjee S, Bhattacharya N, Tripathi A. Differential genotypic signatures of Toll-like receptor polymorphisms among dengue-chikungunya mono- and co-infected Eastern Indian patients.

Eur J Clin Microbiol Infect Dis 2021; 40(7): 1369-81.
[http://dx.doi.org/10.1007/s10096-020-04125-x] [PMID: 33495940]

[9] Valdés-López JF, Fernandez GJ, Urcuqui-Inchima S. Synergistic Effects of Toll-Like Receptor 1/2 and Toll-Like Receptor 3 Signaling Triggering Interleukin 27 Gene Expression in Chikungunya Virus-Infected Macrophages. Front Cell Dev Biol 2022; 10: 812110.
[http://dx.doi.org/10.3389/fcell.2022.812110] [PMID: 35223841]

[10] Mukherjee S, Dutta SK, Sengupta S, Tripathi A. Evidence of dengue and chikungunya virus co-infection and circulation of multiple dengue serotypes in a recent Indian outbreak. Eur J Clin Microbiol Infect Dis 2017; 36(11): 2273-9.
[http://dx.doi.org/10.1007/s10096-017-3061-1] [PMID: 28756561]

[11] Zaidi MB, Garcia-Cordero J, Rivero-Gomez R, *et al.* Competitive suppression of dengue virus replication occurs in chikungunya and dengue co-infected Mexican infants. Parasit Vectors 2018; 11(1): 378.
[http://dx.doi.org/10.1186/s13071-018-2942-1] [PMID: 29970133]

[12] Kashyap RS, Morey S, Bhullar S, *et al.* Determination of Toll-like receptor-induced cytokine profiles in the blood and cerebrospinal fluid of Chikungunya patients. Neuroimmunomodulation 2014; 21(6): 338-46.
[http://dx.doi.org/10.1159/000358240] [PMID: 24776821]

[13] Dutta SK, Tripathi A. Association of toll-like receptor polymorphisms with susceptibility to chikungunya virus infection. Virology 2017; 511: 207-13.
[http://dx.doi.org/10.1016/j.virol.2017.08.009] [PMID: 28888110]

[14] Bucardo F, Reyes Y, Morales M, *et al.* Association of Genetic Polymorphisms in DC-SIGN, Toll-Like Receptor 3, and Tumor Necrosis Factor α Genes and the Lewis-Negative Phenotype With Chikungunya Infection and Disease in Nicaragua. J Infect Dis 2021; 223(2): 278-86.
[http://dx.doi.org/10.1093/infdis/jiaa364] [PMID: 33535235]

[15] Avendaño-Tamayo E, Rúa A, Parra-Marín MV, *et al.* Evaluation of variants in IL6R, TLR3, and DC-SIGN genes associated with dengue in sampled Colombian population. Biomedica 2019; 39(1): 88-101.
[http://dx.doi.org/10.7705/biomedica.v39i1.4029]

[16] Her Z, Teng TS, Tan JJL, *et al.* Loss of TLR3 aggravates CHIKV replication and pathology due to an altered virus-specific neutralizing antibody response. EMBO Mol Med 2015; 7(1): 24-41.
[http://dx.doi.org/10.15252/emmm.201404459] [PMID: 25452586]

[17] Li YG, Siripanyaphinyo U, Tumkosit U, *et al.* Poly (I:C), an agonist of toll-like receptor-3, inhibits replication of the Chikungunya virus in BEAS-2B cells. Virol J 2012; 9(1): 114.
[http://dx.doi.org/10.1186/1743-422X-9-114] [PMID: 22698190]

[18] Fernández-Mestre M, Rauseo DM. X-linked Toll-like receptor 7 polymorphism associated with susceptibility to Chikungunya Fever. Asian Pac J Trop Med 2019; 12(3): 137-41.
[http://dx.doi.org/10.4103/1995-7645.254940]

[19] Lewthwaite P, Vasanthapuram R, Osborne JC, *et al.* Chikungunya virus and central nervous system infections in children, India. Emerg Infect Dis 2009; 15(2): 329-31.
[http://dx.doi.org/10.3201/eid1502.080902]

[20] Grivard P, Le Roux K, Laurent P, *et al.* Molecular and serological diagnosis of Chikungunya virus infection. Pathol Biol (Paris) 2007; 55(10): 490-4.
[http://dx.doi.org/10.1016/j.patbio.2007.07.002]

[21] De Almeida Oliveira Evangelista G, Hughes Carvalho R, Sant'Ana Menezes G, Carvalho de Abreu Y, Sardi SI, Soares Campos G. Meningoencephalitis Associated with Zika Virus and Chikungunya Virus Infection. Jpn J Infect Dis 2021; 74(6): 584-6.
[http://dx.doi.org/10.7883/yoken.JJID.2020.1000]

[22] Carrillo-Hernández MY, Ruiz-Saenz J, Villamizar LJ, Gómez-Rangel SY, Martínez-Gutierrez M. Co-circulation and simultaneous co-infection of dengue, chikungunya, and zika viruses in patients with febrile syndrome at the Colombian-Venezuelan border. BMC Infect Dis 2018; 18(1): 61. [http://dx.doi.org/10.1186/s12879-018-2976-1]

[23] de Souza Costa MC, Siqueira Maia LM, Costa de Souza V, *et al.* Arbovirus investigation in patients from Mato Grosso during Zika and Chikungunya virus introdution in Brazil, 2015-2016. Acta Trop 2019; 190: 395-402. [http://dx.doi.org/10.1016/j.actatropica.2018.12.019]

[24] Mercado-Reyes M, Acosta-Reyes J, Navarro-Lechuga E, *et al.* Dengue, chikungunya and zika virus coinfection: results of the national surveillance during the zika epidemic in Colombia. Epidemiol Infect 2019; 147e77 [http://dx.doi.org/10.1017/S095026881800359X]

[25] Silva MMO, Tauro LB, Kikuti M, *et al.* Concomitant Transmission of Dengue, Chikungunya, and Zika Viruses in Brazil: Clinical and Epidemiological Findings From Surveillance for Acute Febrile Illness. Clin Infect Dis 2019; 69(8): 1353-9. [Erratum in: Clin Infect Dis. 2019 Nov 27;69]. [12]. [:2238. Erratum in: Clin Infect Dis. 2019 Nov 27;69]. [12]. [:2238. PMID: 30561554; PMCID: PMC7348233]. [http://dx.doi.org/10.1093/cid/ciy1083]

[26] Stanley J, Chongkolwatana V, Duong PT, *et al.* Detection of dengue, chikungunya, and Zika RNA in blood donors from Southeast Asia. Transfusion 2021; 61(1): 134-43. [http://dx.doi.org/10.1111/trf.16110]

[27] Pavon JAR, Neves NADS, Silva LCF, *et al.* Neurological infection by chikungunya and a triple Arbovirus co-infection in Mato Grosso, Central Western Brazil during 2019. J Clin Virol 2022; 146105056 [http://dx.doi.org/10.1016/j.jcv.2021.105056]

[28] de Souza TMA, Ribeiro ED, Corrêa VCE, *et al.* Following in the Footsteps of the Chikungunya Virus in Brazil: The First Autochthonous Cases in Amapá in 2014 and Its Emergence in Rio de Janeiro during 2016. Viruses 2018; 10(11): 623. [http://dx.doi.org/10.3390/v10110623]

[29] Saswat T, Kumar A, Kumar S, *et al.* High rates of co-infection of Dengue and Chikungunya virus in Odisha and Maharashtra, India during 2013. Infect Genet Evol 2015; 35: 134-41. [http://dx.doi.org/10.1016/j.meegid.2015.08.006]

[30] Hisamuddin M, Tazeen A, Abdullah M, *et al.* Co-circulation of Chikungunya and Dengue viruses in Dengue endemic region of New Delhi, India during 2016. Epidemiol Infect 2018; 146(13): 1642-53. [http://dx.doi.org/10.1017/S0950268818001590]

[31] Afreen N, Deeba F, Khan WH, *et al.* Molecular characterization of dengue and chikungunya virus strains circulating in New Delhi, India. Microbiol Immunol 2014; 58(12): 688-96. [http://dx.doi.org/10.1111/1348-0421.12209]

[32] Jain J, Okabayashi T, Kaur N, *et al.* Evaluation of an immunochromatography rapid diagnosis kit for detection of chikungunya virus antigen in India, a dengue-endemic country. Virol J 2018; 15(1): 84. [http://dx.doi.org/10.1186/s12985-018-1000-0]

[33] Myint KSA, Mawuntu AHP, Haryanto S, *et al.* Neurological Disease Associated with Chikungunya in Indonesia. Am J Trop Med Hyg 2022; 107(2): 291-5. Epub ahead of print [http://dx.doi.org/10.4269/ajtmh.22-0050]

CHAPTER 8

West Nile Virus and Toll-like Receptors

Abstract: West Nile Fever is transmitted by West Nile Virus (WNV), which is a single-stranded RNS *flavivirus*. This disease is transmitted by the bite of mosquitoes. This disease is endemic in various countries in Africa, Asia, Europe and North America [1, 2]. There is no vaccine yet for this disease which is displayed by various symptoms in humans varying from neurological squealae (encephalitis) and meningitis. Apart from this, patients report fever, headache, and myalgia as well.

Keywords: MicroRNAs, MyD88, Myeloid differentiation factor 88-deficient (*Myd88*$^{-/-}$), NF-κB, STAT1, TRAF3.

INTRODUCTION

TLRs 7 and 3 can act to prevent or aggravate the pathogenicity of WNV infection. TLR3 depended on promoted entry of WNV in brain pathogenesis followed by neuronal injury in mice [3]. On the other hand, it was demonstrated that there was no difference in the susceptibility of Mice to WNV in TLR-/- and wild-type mice [4].

To effective WNV clearance upon infection, TLR7 and IL23 intact condition is required. However, TLR7 -/- and myeloid differentiation factor 88-deficient (*Myd88*$^{-/-}$) mice failed to detect the WNV which lead to a further increase of viremia causing the susceptibility [5]. The resident tissue macrophages such as kupffer cells in the liver and microglia in the brain, sense the WNV by TLR and through the IL-23 signalling pathway they recruit more immune cells to the infected organs. This mechanism is compromised in TLR7-/- mice leading to high viremia. This TLR7 and IL23 interaction are necessary for immune cell homing to the affected /infected cells, thus pharmacotherapy can consider these molecules for a therapeutic approach to WNV infection.

West Nile virus was infected in equine PBMCs and was analyzed for the presence of TLR signature. The findings revealed the upregulation of TLR1, 3, 5, 7-9 transcripts followed by TRAF3, MyD88, STAT1, NF-κB, and 2, ISG15, IRF3, and 7, SOCS1, and 3 in the infected cells in comparison with the control cells [6]. Stingingly, post-infection of 24 hrs raised the viral titer in the cells but further

Jayalakshmi Krishnan

replication of the virus was stopped in the subsequent hours. The rise of the TLR genes and their subsequent signal transduction proteins could be the reason why the replication of the virus was not noted after 24 hrs in equine PBMCs [6].

TLR8 is not explored properly for its role in WNV infection. A study found that the TLR8-/- murine cells were resistant to the WNV infection [7, 8]. TLR7 mediates antiviral responses against WNV. Overexpression of *TLR7* and IFN-stimulated gene-56 expression was observed in TLR8-/- mice. This overexpression of *TLR7* has caused the effective clearance of the WNV virus. SOCS 1 is associated with TLR8 and not with TLR7, the selective knockdown of SOCS 1 resulted in higher IFN responses followed by *TLR7*expression [7, 8]. These findings clearly indicate that TLR8 is blocking the expression of TLR7-mediated WNV clearance and anti-viral responses by coupling with SOCS1.

Human studies on WNV infection and the responses of the primary human macrophages have shown surprising findings. In humans, the elderly are very prone to WNV infection causing death in them due to poor immune responses. When the primary human macrophages of the elderly and young donors after MWN infection were investigated it was found that there were higher TLR3 levels and cytokine levels in the elderly than in the young donor cells [9]. This is due to the presence of a signal transducer and activator of the transcription 1 (STAT1)-mediated pathway. Glycosylated WNV envelope protein from WNV upon binding with C-type lectin dendritic cell-specific intercellular adhesion molecule 3 (ICAM3) and DC-SIGN cause the downregulation of TLR3 this is mediated *via* STAT1. In elderly patients, there is a cytokine storm due to the high levels of TLR3 and it leads to blood-brain barrier disruption which causes these brain infections of WNV.

MicroRNAs and West Nile Virus

MicroRNAs have been investigated and found to be very reliable biomarkers for TLR activation. A study has been conducted in HEK293-NULL and HEK293-TLR3 cells infected with WNV to understand the pattern of innate immune responses. NF-kB gene signature revealed that TLR3 was solemnly responsible for WNV-induced gene signature. The study further explored the miRNA expression events in the TLR3 knockout condition. There were 70 microRNAs produced upon WNV infection *via* TLR3 signaling. These microRNAs were found to be involved in regulating cell death, viral pathogenesis, and immune cell trafficking [10].

TLR3 participates actively in triggering the pathogenesis of the West Nile Virus. In the brain, the neuronal injury to the WNV is caused by the leaking of blood-brain barrier by the activation of TNFa produced *via* TLR3 [3, 11]. TLR3 seems to do cross-priming of immune cells, which plays an important role in CD8+ T cell responses to proteins. TLR3 activation is a must for the antigen-presenting cells such as dendritic cells to act, as this activation increases the phagocytosis of infected material [12]. In the CNS, the knockout of TLR3 and the intracranial injection of WNV caused increased viral replication in primary cortical neurons [13].

MyD88-/- and TLR-/- and WNV infection

When compared to wild type mice MyD88/Trif−/− displayed high viral burden leading to increased susceptibility to the virus [14]. Inflammatory events, microglail activation and astrogliosis were also witnessed due to high viral burden [14]. TLR3 and microRNAs role have been investigated in the WNV infection in HEK293-NULL and HEK293-TLR3 cells.In a TLR3 independent manner microRNAs (70 of them) have been induced which are responsible for cell death, immune cell trafficking and viral pathogenesis [15]. Upon investigation with TLR7-/- and MyD88 deficient mice after WNV infection they had reduced interleukin responses [16]. TLR3-/- mice is investigated for its role in west nile virus infection.In primary cortical neuronal cultures this deficiency of TLR3 is causing enhanced viral replication. In CNS tissues deficiency of IRF 7 leads to increased viral load and also in various cells such as cortical neurons, DCs, fibroblasts, and macrophages [17]. Various TLRs mRNA were increased along with signalling pathway genes in equine cells upon exposure to west nile virus infection [18]. There are studies which prove that genetically knockout conditions with TLRs to WNV, has increased viral load and increased susceptibility to the infection [19 - 22]. Not only TLRs but RLRs pathways are also involved in controlling the infections caused by WNV [23]. Following intradermal injection of WNV in TLR7-/- mice, Langerhans cells were reduced not in TLR7 minus mice but in wild type mice. Even the infection with WNV was higher in keratinocytes of TLR7 minus than the wild type keratinocytes. TLR7 modulates the expression of various cells in the body by that it can contribute to the systemic infection [24]. In old (21- to 22-month) mice the susceptibility to WNV virus was assessed in comparition with young (6- to 10-week-old) mice. Impaired TLR signalling in old mice contributes to the loss of innate and adaptive immune system that lead to susceptibility to the virus [25]. NS4B-P38G mutant west nile virus was investigated in the MyD88 -/- and TLR7 -/-mice and it was found that they were more susceptible than the wild type mice [26]. Upon WNV infection, TLR3 knockout mice were very much resistant to the virus. Not only resistant but it also has increased viral load in various tissues including brain causing neuropathological changes [27]. When exposed to west nile virus, TLR3-/- neuronal cells were showing increased expression in comparison with wild type cells upon west nile virus infection. Further, there was increased viral burden was noted in TLR3 -/- cells in comparison with wild type cells [28 - 30]. High viral yields were seen in the human brain glioma cells exposed to west nile virus infection followed by cytopathologic effects [31]. In these cells, innate immune responses were created by type I interferon pathways which leads to the activation of gial cells. These glail cell activation leads to the phagocyte activity against the virus. However in some cross bread mouse models it is reported that T cells restrict the immune responses thus contributing to the persisting of infection in CNS for long time [32]. There are studies in mice which prove that inoculation of west nile virus to the footpad of the mouse will get the mouse infected and kill the mouse within 10-12 days [33 - 35]. Neurodegeneration caused by west nile virus is often due to production of interferons, interleukins and alpha sinucleins followed by activation of ubiquitin signalled protein activation. From the skin after infection the west nile virus spreads to the lymph nodes. The route of entry of WNV to the brain seems to be mediated by various methods such as breaking the brain parenchyma, breakdown of the blood brain barrier, transendothelial spread and transsynaptic spread. However all strains of the virus may not follow all these kind of the pathways to enter the CNS but it may vary from strain to strain.

WNV replication occurs in the cytoplasm of the infected cells. WNV has both structural and non-structural proteins, there are three structural proteins namely C, prM/M, and E for the virus attachment and entry. There are seven non structural proteins named as NS1, NS2A, NS2B, NS3, NS4A, NS4B, and NS5 responsible for viral RNA synthesis. The Toll like receptors and also the RIG I like receptors along with Nod like receptor sense and detect WNV to elicit innate immune responses. Compared to wild type mice, *ST*imulator of *IN*terferon *G*ene (STING) STING-/- mice, has shown severe neurological sequences .If the virus crosses the blood brain barrier it leads to most serious case known as West Nile Neuroinvasive Disease (WNND) [36]. This disease is characterised by gastric complications, Parkinson's like termers, encephalitis and meningitis [37 - 39]. The performance of the recovery of patients from WNV even after 18 months is displaying minor cognitive decline [39]. WNV associated retinopathy is reported to be present in 24% of the patients who are infected with the virus [40]. This retinopathy is observed in patients with neurological impairments. The cognitive deficits associated with WNV infection is irrespective of the virus infection such as WNV or West Nile Neuroinvasive Disease (WNND).These cognitive deficits are more prevalent with increasing days of infection [41].

Permanent damage to central nervous system causes persistent cognitive impairment in patients even after one year of infection in Mexico [42]. In a telephonic interview conducted between the patients (116 of them) of west Nile fever and or west Nile neuroinvasive diseases it was seen that the mental status was very poor and there was decline in cognitive skills [43]. Studies in Greece in 2010 has reported that there was a noninvasive WNV infection characterised by leukopenia, Rashes, Myalgia and febrile nature [44]. There was outbreak of WNV cases in Greece between July and August 2011, as 17 cases out of 31 infections were reported from those areas where the disease was not reported previously [45]. 14 Culex spp. pools were collected from a province in Greece showing H249P substitution in the NS3 protein with two different lineages [46]. WNV infection is also seen in New York city in 1999, with 59 patients admitted mostly in elderly patients above 71 years of old [47]. There was a dysfunction of T cells in WNV that leads to disease severity. Human macrophage derived dendrite cells were stopped by the WNV infection thus leading to less inflammatory responses [48]. In USA Illinois state reported 21% of WNV cases in 2002 with elderly patients being much affected [49]. Among the follow up of one year after the WNV infection cases in the state of Louisiana it is reported that it has affected mind and body [50].

Human dendritic cells when infected with WNV reduce the interaction of DC- and invariant natural killer cells leading to less proinflammatory molecules [51]. Gamma dendrite cell deficient mice displayed lower levels of CD molecules such as CD40, CD80, CD86 and MHC class II less expression. On the other hand WNV infected gamma delta cells induces DC maturation thus causes CD4(+) T-cell priming [52]. There are two types of gamma T cells, Vgamma1(+) and Vgamma4(+) cells they play a differential role in host cell immunity to WNV. Mice without Vgamma1(+) cells have displayed high viral loads and higher mortality to the WNV.On the other hand mice lacking Vgamma4(+) cells display reductions in TNF alpha levels followed by lower mortality and less viral load in brain [53]. There are other type of cells called as Vγ4(+) cells, which are involved in the pathogenesis of WNV. In mice lacking Vγ4(+) cells infected with WNV low viremia and reductions in the inflammatory responses were observed [54]. Brain infiltrated lymphocytes is known to play very important role in the pathogenesis of west nile virus infection. In mice infected with WNV it is known that TCR alpha chain play an important role in the T cells. CD3(+)CD8(+) T cells were seen in the mice infected brains infected with WNV. CD8(+) T cells infiltrating T cells are specific to WNV and they are not having cross reactivity [55].

There was an increase in CD3, CD8, CD25, and CD69 molecules in JEV infected mice. The differences in the incoming T cells determine the fate of the JEV infected mice whether it can survive or die [56]. $CD8^+$ T cells such as $PD1^+CCR2^+CD8^+$ T cells is known to infiltrate the Central nervous system of the mice leading to the pathogenecity of the virus [57]. Chemokines like CCR5 induces the infiltration or migration of NK cells, macrophages and T cells into the tissues .By facilitating the infiltration of T regulatory cells CD4(+)Foxp3(+) in to the CNS these CCR5 molecules facilitate the mice survival [58].

TCRdelta(-/-) mice have higher viral loads and cause increased pathogenecity of the virus to the central nervous system [59]. Gammadelta T cells seems to curb the spread of WNV infection by enhancing the adaptive immune responses. 15% of TCRdelta(-/-) mice [60]. Two cycles of stimulation of T and B cells are needed in older mice to elicit both cellular and adaptive immunity against the WNV [61].CD4 + cells act independantly in protecting the C57BL/6 (H-2(b)) mice, infected with WNV than the B cells and CD8 T cells [62]. However role of CD8 cells also was investigated and found that naïve CD8(+)T cells transfer after high enrichment shows that WNV infected mice is protected. This clearly indicates that CD8 + cells alone can protect the mice from the WNV [63].Defective CD8 and CD4 cells caused death in the WNV infected old mice in comparison with wild types mice [64].Role of CD40 ligand was also investigated in WNV infection. CD40(-/-) mice are vulnerable to WNV infection and die.

WNV-specific immunoglobulin M (IgM) and IgG, levels were very low in the mice which lack CD40(-/-). Also these CD40 ligand interactions causes the migration of the CD8+ T cells in the brain of the mice leading to the protection from the virus [65]. Also, WNV clearing in mice is mediated by CD4+ T cells during primary viral infections as these cells sustain the CD8 + T cells which help in clearing the pathogen [66].

MDA 5 is pattern recognition receptor MDA5(-/-) mice were highly vulnerable to the infection and showed defects in the central nervous system of the mice. The immune priming is done by MDA 5 by which the CD8 T cell is activated and migrates to CNS to clear the infection [67]. In cell culture setting its is shown that Tumor necrosis factor-related apoptosis-inducing ligand can inhibit the *flaviviruses*. In TRAIL(-/-) mice, upon WNV infection T cells struggle to clear the infection. However, CD8 T cells which produce TRAIL clear the WNV from neurons [68]. WNV infection triggers the T cells to produce perforin of FAS to clear the infection. In lineage I New York isolate of WNV infection in mice, defective perforin leads to higher viral titer and caused the death of the mice [69].

CD8 T cells express Fas-Fas ligand (FasL) with causes the clearance of the WNNV infection from mice (70). 100% mortality was seen in the mice with IFN-alpha/beta receptor-deficiency exposed to WNV infection causing the death of the animal [71]. Interferon gamma plays an important role in the viral clearance. IFN-gamma(-/-) and IFN-gammaR(-/-) upon WNV infection showed high viral load and increased reduced survival time and 90%of the mice died [72].Knocking out TLR7 and MyD88 in mice can enhance the susceptibility of the mice to the WN virus by leading to high viral load in liver, spleen and blood of the mice [73]. There are 5 types of lineages for west nile virus out of which first two lineages that is I and II have been properly investigated and understood it has spread its tentacles from Africa to Europe [74].

In 1999 the outbreak of WNV in New York city was caused by Lineage I and since then there are two types of strains are also identified such as NY99 strain and WN02 strain [75, 76]. Upon infection with west nile virus in the brain, it is seen that macrophages are invading and causing the inflammation. This macrophage act as antigen presenting cells and in mice the antiviral responses are mediated by TLR3 by activated microglial cells [77 - 79]. One subset of T cells known as γδd T cells causes the expansion of dendritic cells to produce enormous amount of IFN gamma [80].There are studies which point out that in a TLR3 independent manner 70 microRNAs are produced in HEK29 cells upon infection with west nile virus [81].Apart from TLRs as pattern recognition receptors RIGI and MDA 5 act also as pattern recognition receptors in defence against the West nile virus.

In fibroblasts derived from wild type and RIG I null mice have shown that the inflammatory responses were delayed in the RIGI null mice [82]. However, on the other hand it was shown that there is antognosit action by NS1 protein of WNV to Interferon beta production by nullifying the action of RIGi-RLR activation [83]. mice null in TLR7 and MyD88 fail to recognize ssRNA, with high viremia and higher susceptibility to the west nile virus .Even the presence of CD5 and CD11 macrophages could not present the infected cells in the mice devoid of TLR7 [84]. Similarly in comparison with wild type mice, MyD88/Trif-/- mice display higher susceptibility to west nile virus infection with elevated cell infiltration [85].

CONCLUDING REMARKS

WNV infection causes severe infection in humans. Through the adaptor molecule TRIF and MyD88 the signals are generated from TLRs upon WNV binding to initiate innate immune signaling to fight the virus. Non-structural proteins from the west nile virus can inhibit the TLR3-mediated signal transduction. Through TLR3 type I Interferons are produced. In the CNS it was shown that TLR3 is involved in protection from the west nile virus. TLR3 -/- mice are shown to produce less TNF alpha levels and interleukin levels. Upon WNV infection higher levels of TLRs were seen in PBMCs, particularly TLR3,4, and 6 levels.

CONSENT FOR PUBLICATION

Not applicable.

CONFLICT OF INTEREST

The author declares no conflict of interest, financial or otherwise.

ACKNOWLEDGEMENT

Declared none.

REFERENCES

[1] Valdés-López JF, Velilla P, Urcuqui-Inchima S. Vitamin D modulates the expression of Toll-like receptors and pro-inflammatory cytokines without affecting Chikungunya virus replication, in monocytes and macrophages. Acta Trop 2022; 232(1): 106497. [http://dx.doi.org/10.1016/j.actatropica.2022.106497] [PMID: 35508271]

[2] Pletnev AG, Swayne DE, Speicher J, Rumyantsev AA, Murphy BR. Chimeric West Nile/dengue virus vaccine candidate: Preclinical evaluation in mice, geese and monkeys for safety and immunogenicity. Vaccine 2006; 24(40-41): 6392-404. [http://dx.doi.org/10.1016/j.vaccine.2006.06.008] [PMID: 16831498]

[3] Wang T, Town T, Alexopoulou L, Anderson JF, Fikrig E, Flavell RA. Toll-like receptor 3 mediates West Nile virus entry into the brain causing lethal encephalitis. Nat Med 2004; 10(12): 1366-73. [http://dx.doi.org/10.1038/nm1140] [PMID: 15558055]

[4] Welte T, Reagan K, Fang H, *et al.* Toll-like receptor 7-induced immune response to cutaneous West Nile virus infection. J Gen Virol 2009; 90(11): 2660-8. [http://dx.doi.org/10.1099/vir.0.011783-0] [PMID: 19641044]

[5] Town T, Bai F, Wang T, *et al.* Toll-like receptor 7 mitigates lethal West Nile encephalitis *via* interleukin 23-dependent immune cell infiltration and homing. Immunity 2009; 30(2): 242-53. [http://dx.doi.org/10.1016/j.immuni.2008.11.012] [PMID: 19200759]

[6] Uddin MJ, Suen WW, Bosco-Lauth A, *et al.* Kinetics of the West Nile virus induced transcripts of selected cytokines and Toll-like receptors in equine peripheral blood mononuclear cells. Vet Res 2016; 47(1): 61. [http://dx.doi.org/10.1186/s13567-016-0347-8] [PMID: 27267361]

[7] Paul AM, Acharya D, Le L, *et al.* TLR8 couples SOCS-1 and restrains TLR7-mediated antiviral immunity, exacerbating West Nile virus infection in mice. J Immunol 2016; 197(11): 4425-35. [http://dx.doi.org/10.4049/jimmunol.1600902] [PMID: 27798161]

[8] Halliday A, Bates PA, Chance ML, Taylor MJ. Toll-like receptor 2 (TLR2) plays a role in controlling cutaneous leishmaniasis *in vivo*, but does not require activation by parasite lipophosphoglycan. Parasit Vectors 2016; 9(1): 532. [http://dx.doi.org/10.1186/s13071-016-1807-8] [PMID: 27716391]

[9] Kong KF, Delroux K, Wang X, *et al.* Dysregulation of TLR3 impairs the innate immune response to West Nile virus in the elderly. J Virol 2008; 82(15): 7613-23. [http://dx.doi.org/10.1128/JVI.00618-08] [PMID: 18508883]

[10] Chugh PE, Damania BA, Dittmer DP. Toll-like receptor-3 is dispensable for the innate microRNA response to West Nile virus (WNV). PLoS One 2014; 9(8): e104770. [http://dx.doi.org/10.1371/journal.pone.0104770] [PMID: 25127040]

[11] Diamond MS, Klein RS. West Nile virus: crossing the blood-brain barrier. Nat Med 2004; 10(12): 1294-5. [http://dx.doi.org/10.1038/nm1204-1294] [PMID: 15580248]

[12] Schulz O, Diebold SS, Chen M, *et al.* Toll-like receptor 3 promotes cross-priming to virus-infected cells. Nature 2005; 433(7028): 887-92.

[http://dx.doi.org/10.1038/nature03326] [PMID: 15711573]

[13] Daffis S, Samuel MA, Suthar MS, Gale M Jr, Diamond MS. Toll-like receptor 3 has a protective role against West Nile virus infection. J Virol 2008; 82(21): 10349-58. [http://dx.doi.org/10.1128/JVI.00935-08] [PMID: 18715906]

[14] Sabouri AH, Marcondes MCG, Flynn C, *et al.* TLR signaling controls lethal encephalitis in WNV-infected brain. Brain Res 2014; 1574: 84-95. [http://dx.doi.org/10.1016/j.brainres.2014.05.049] [PMID: 24928618]

[15] Chugh PE, Damania BA, Dittmer DP. Toll-like receptor-3 is dispensable for the innate microRNA response to West Nile virus (WNV). PLoS One 2014; 9(8): e104770. [http://dx.doi.org/10.1371/journal.pone.0104770] [PMID: 25127040]

[16] Town T, Bai F, Wang T, *et al.* Toll-like receptor 7 mitigates lethal West Nile encephalitis *via* interleukin 23-dependent immune cell infiltration and homing. Immunity 2009; 30(2): 242-53. [http://dx.doi.org/10.1016/j.immuni.2008.11.012] [PMID: 19200759]

[17] Daffis S, Samuel MA, Suthar MS, Keller BC, Gale M Jr, Diamond MS. Interferon regulatory factor IRF-7 induces the antiviral alpha interferon response and protects against lethal West Nile virus infection. J Virol 2008; 82(17): 8465-75. [http://dx.doi.org/10.1128/JVI.00918-08] [PMID: 18562536]

[18] Uddin MJ, Suen WW, Bosco-Lauth A, *et al.* Kinetics of the West Nile virus induced transcripts of selected cytokines and Toll-like receptors in equine peripheral blood mononuclear cells. Vet Res 2016; 47(1): 61. [http://dx.doi.org/10.1186/s13567-016-0347-8] [PMID: 27267361]

[19] Durrant DM, Robinette ML, Klein RS. IL-1R1 is required for dendritic cell–mediated T cell reactivation within the CNS during West Nile virus encephalitis. J Exp Med 2013; 210(3): 503-16. [http://dx.doi.org/10.1084/jem.20121897] [PMID: 23460727]

[20] Ramos HJ, Lanteri MC, Blahnik G, *et al.* IL-1β signaling promotes CNS-intrinsic immune control of West Nile virus infection. PLoS Pathog 2012; 8(11): e1003039. [http://dx.doi.org/10.1371/journal.ppat.1003039] [PMID: 23209411]

[21] Town T, Bai F, Wang T, *et al.* Toll-like receptor 7 mitigates lethal West Nile encephalitis *via* interleukin 23-dependent immune cell infiltration and homing. Immunity 2009; 30(2): 242-53. [http://dx.doi.org/10.1016/j.immuni.2008.11.012] [PMID: 19200759]

[22] Town T, Bai F, Wang T, *et al.* Toll-like receptor 7 mitigates lethal West Nile encephalitis *via* interleukin 23-dependent immune cell infiltration and homing. Immunity 2009; 30(2): 242-53. [http://dx.doi.org/10.1016/j.immuni.2008.11.012] [PMID: 19200759]

[23] Suthar MS, Ma DY, Thomas S, *et al.* IPS-1 is essential for the control of West Nile virus infection and immunity. PLoS Pathog 2010; 6(2): e1000757. [http://dx.doi.org/10.1371/journal.ppat.1000757] [PMID: 20140199]

[24] Welte T, Reagan K, Fang H, *et al.* Toll-like receptor 7-induced immune response to cutaneous West Nile virus infection. J Gen Virol 2009; 90(11): 2660-8. [http://dx.doi.org/10.1099/vir.0.011783-0] [PMID: 19641044]

[25] Xie G, Luo H, Pang L, *et al.* Dysregulation of toll-like receptor 7 compromises innate and adaptive T cell responses and host resistance to an attenuated west nile virus infection in old mice. J Virol 2016; 90(3): 1333-44. [http://dx.doi.org/10.1128/JVI.02488-15] [PMID: 26581984]

[26] Xie G, Welte T, Wang J, *et al.* A West Nile virus NS4B-P38G mutant strain induces adaptive immunity *via* TLR7-MyD88-dependent and independent signaling pathways. Vaccine 2013; 31(38): 4143-51. [http://dx.doi.org/10.1016/j.vaccine.2013.06.093] [PMID: 23845800]

[27] Wang T, Town T, Alexopoulou L, Anderson JF, Fikrig E, Flavell RA. Toll-like receptor 3 mediates

West Nile virus entry into the brain causing lethal encephalitis. Nat Med 2004; 10(12): 1366-73. [http://dx.doi.org/10.1038/nm1140] [PMID: 15558055]

[28] Zhou Y, Ye L, Wan Q, *et al.* Activation of Toll-like receptors inhibits herpes simplex virus-1 infection of human neuronal cells. J Neurosci Res 2009; 87(13): 2916-25. [http://dx.doi.org/10.1002/jnr.22110] [PMID: 19437550]

[29] Zhou L, Wang X, Wang YJ, *et al.* Activation of Toll-like receptor-3 induces interferon-λ expression in human neuronal cells. Neuroscience 2009; 159(2): 629-37. [http://dx.doi.org/10.1016/j.neuroscience.2008.12.036] [PMID: 19166911]

[30] Piersanti S, Astrologo L, Licursi V, *et al.* Differentiated neuroprogenitor cells incubated with human or canine adenovirus, or lentiviral vectors have distinct transcriptome profiles. PLoS One 2013; 8(7): e69808. [http://dx.doi.org/10.1371/journal.pone.0069808] [PMID: 23922808]

[31] Koh WL, Ng ML. Molecular mechanisms of West Nile virus pathogenesis in brain cell. Emerg Infect Dis 2005; 11(4): 629-32. [http://dx.doi.org/10.3201/eid1104.041076]

[32] Graham JB, Swarts JL, Wilkins C, Thomas S, Green R, Sekine A, *et al.* A Mouse Model of Chronic West Nile Virus Disease. PLoS Pathog 2016; 12(11)e1005996 [http://dx.doi.org/10.1371/journal.ppat.1005996]

[33] Daffis S, Samuel MA, Keller BC, Gale M Jr, Diamond MS. Cell-specific IRF-3 responses protect against West Nile virus infection by interferon-dependent and -independent mechanisms. PLoS Pathog 2007; 3e106

[34] Daffis S, Samuel MA, Suthar MS, Gale M Jr, Diamond MS. Toll-like receptor 3 has a protective role against West Nile virus infection. J Virol 2008; 82: 10349-58.

[35] Daffis S, Samuel MA, Suthar MS, *et al.* Interferon regulatory factor IRF-7 induces the antiviral alpha interferon response and protects against lethal West Nile virus infection. J Virol 2008; 82: 8465-75.

[36] Sejvar JJ, Haddad MB, Tierney BC, Campbell GL, Marfin AA, Van Gerpen JA, *et al.* Neurologic manifestations and outcome of West Nile virus infection. JAMA 2003; 290(4): 511-5.

[37] Sejvar JJ, Haddad MB, Tierney BC, Campbell GL, Marfin AA, Van Gerpen JA, *et al.* Neurologic manifestations and outcome of West Nile virus infection. JAMA 2003; 290(4): 511-5.

[38] Sejvar JJ, Curns AT, Welburg L, Jones JF, Lundgren LM, Capuron L, *et al.* Neurocognitive and functional outcomes in persons recovering from West Nile virus illness. J Neuropsychol 2008; 2(Pt 2): 477-99.

[39] Russo MV, McGavern DB. Immune Surveillance of the CNS following Infection and Injury. Trends Immunol 2015; 36(10): 637-50.

[40] Hasbun R, Garcia MN, Kellaway J, *et al.* West Nile Virus Retinopathy and Associations with Long Term Neurological and Neurocognitive Sequelae. PLoS One 2016; 11(3)e0148898 [http://dx.doi.org/10.1371/journal.pone.0148898]

[41] Samaan Z, McDermid Vaz S, Bawor M, Potter TH, Eskandarian S, Loeb M. Neuropsychological Impact of West Nile Virus Infection: An Extensive Neuropsychiatric Assessment of 49 Cases in Canada. PLoS One 2016; 11(6)e0158364 [http://dx.doi.org/10.1371/journal.pone.0158364]

[42] Sadek JR, Pergam SA, Harrington JA, *et al.* Persistent neuropsychological impairment associated with West Nile virus infection. J Clin Exp Neuropsychol 2010; 32(1): 81-7. [http://dx.doi.org/10.1080/13803390902881918]

[43] Haaland KY, Sadek J, Pergam S, *et al.* Mental status after West Nile virus infection. Emerg Infect Dis 2006; 12(8): 1260-2. [http://dx.doi.org/10.3201/eid1708.060097]

[44] Anastasiadou A, Economopoulou A, Kakoulidis I, *et al.* Non-neuroinvasive West Nile virus infections during the outbreak in Greece. Clin Microbiol Infect 2011; 17(11): 1681-3. [http://dx.doi.org/10.1111/j.1469-0691.2011.03642.x]

[45] Danis K, Papa A, Papanikolaou E, *et al.* Ongoing outbreak of West Nile virus infection in humans, Greece, July to August 2011. Euro Surveill 2011; 16(34): 19951.

[46] Papa A, Papadopoulou E, Gavana E, Kalaitzopoulou S, Mourelatos S. Detection of West Nile virus lineage 2 in Culex mosquitoes, Greece, 2012. Vector Borne Zoonotic Dis 2013; 13(9): 682-4. [http://dx.doi.org/10.1089/vbz.2012.1212]

[47] Nash D, Mostashari F, Fine A, *et al.* 1999 West Nile Outbreak Response Working Group. The outbreak of West Nile virus infection in the New York City area in 1999. N Engl J Med 2001; 344(24): 1807-14. [http://dx.doi.org/10.1056/NEJM200106143442401]

[48] Zimmerman MG, Bowen JR, McDonald CE, Pulendran B, Suthar MS. West Nile Virus Infection Blocks Inflammatory Response and T Cell Costimulatory Capacity of Human Monocyte-Derived Dendritic Cells. J Virol 2019; 93(23): e00664-19. [http://dx.doi.org/10.1128/JVI.00664-19]

[49] Huhn GD, Austin C, Langkop C, *et al.* The emergence of west nile virus during a large outbreak in Illinois in 2002. Am J Trop Med Hyg 2005; 72(6): 768-76.

[50] Ou AC, Ratard RC. One-year sequelae in patients with West Nile Virus encephalitis and meningitis in Louisiana. J La State Med Soc 2005; 157(1): 42-6.

[51] Kovats S, Turner S, Simmons A, Powe T, Chakravarty E, Alberola-Ila J. West Nile virus-infected human dendritic cells fail to fully activate invariant natural killer T cells. Clin Exp Immunol 2016; 186(2): 214-26. [http://dx.doi.org/10.1111/cei.12850]

[52] Fang H, Welte T, Zheng X, *et al.* gammadelta T cells promote the maturation of dendritic cells during West Nile virus infection. FEMS Immunol Med Microbiol 2010; 59(1): 71-80. [http://dx.doi.org/10.1111/j.1574-695X.2010.00663.x]

[53] Welte T, Lamb J, Anderson JF, Born WK, O'Brien RL, Wang T. Role of two distinct gammadelta T cell subsets during West Nile virus infection. FEMS Immunol Med Microbiol 2008; 53(2): 275-83. [http://dx.doi.org/10.1111/j.1574-695X.2008.00430.x]

[54] Welte T, Aronson J, Gong B, *et al.* Vγ4+ T cells regulate host immune response to West Nile virus infection. FEMS Immunol Med Microbiol 2011; 63(2): 183-92. [http://dx.doi.org/10.1111/j.1574-695X.2011.00840.x]

[55] Kitaura K, Fujii Y, Hayasaka D, *et al.* High clonality of virus-specific T lymphocytes defined by TCR usage in the brains of mice infected with West Nile virus. J Immunol 2011; 187(8): 3919-30. [http://dx.doi.org/10.4049/jimmunol.1100442]

[56] Shirai K, Hayasaka D, Kitaura K, *et al.* Qualitative differences in brain-infiltrating T cells are associated with a fatal outcome in mice infected with Japanese encephalitis virus. Arch Virol 2015; 160(3): 765-75. [http://dx.doi.org/10.1007/s00705-014-2154-8]

[57] Zhang F, Qi L, Li T, *et al.* $PD1^{+}CCR2^{+}CD8^{+}$ T Cells Infiltrate the Central Nervous System during Acute Japanese Encephalitis Virus Infection. Virol Sin 2019; 34(5): 538-48. [http://dx.doi.org/10.1007/s12250-019-00134-z]

[58] Kim JH, Patil AM, Choi JY, *et al.* CCR5 ameliorates Japanese encephalitis *via* dictating the equilibrium of regulatory CD4(+)Foxp3(+) T and IL-17(+)CD4(+) Th17 cells. J Neuroinflammation 2016; 13(1): 223. [http://dx.doi.org/10.1186/s12974-016-0656-x]

[59] Wang T, Scully E, Yin Z, *et al.* IFN-gamma-producing gamma delta T cells help control murine West Nile virus infection. J Immunol 2003; 171(5): 2524-31. [http://dx.doi.org/10.4049/jimmunol.171.5.2524]

[60] Wang T, Gao Y, Scully E, *et al.* Gamma delta T cells facilitate adaptive immunity against West Nile virus infection in mice. J Immunol 2006; 177(3): 1825-32. [http://dx.doi.org/10.4049/jimmunol.177.3.1825]

[61] Uhrlaub JL, Brien JD, Widman DG, Mason PW, Nikolich-Zugich J. Repeated *in vivo* stimulation of T and B cell responses in old mice generates protective immunity against lethal West Nile virus encephalitis. J Immunol 2011; 186(7): 3882-91. [http://dx.doi.org/10.4049/jimmunol.1002799]

[62] Brien JD, Uhrlaub JL, Nikolich-Zugich J. West Nile virus-specific CD4 T cells exhibit direct antiviral cytokine secretion and cytotoxicity and are sufficient for antiviral protection. J Immunol 2008; 181(12): 8568-75. [http://dx.doi.org/10.4049/jimmunol.181.12.8568]

[63] Brien JD, Uhrlaub JL, Nikolich-Zugich J. Protective capacity and epitope specificity of CD8(+) T cells responding to lethal West Nile virus infection. Eur J Immunol 2007; 37(7): 1855-63. [http://dx.doi.org/10.1002/eji.200737196]

[64] Brien JD, Uhrlaub JL, Hirsch A, Wiley CA, Nikolich-Zugich J. Key role of T cell defects in age-related vulnerability to West Nile virus. J Exp Med 2009; 206(12): 2735-45. [http://dx.doi.org/10.1084/jem.20090222]

[65] Sitati E, McCandless EE, Klein RS, Diamond MS. CD40-CD40 ligand interactions promote trafficking of CD8+ T cells into the brain and protection against West Nile virus encephalitis. J Virol 2007; 81(18): 9801-11. [http://dx.doi.org/10.1128/JVI.00941-07]

[66] Sitati EM, Diamond MS. CD4+ T-cell responses are required for clearance of West Nile virus from the central nervous system. J Virol 2006; 80(24): 12060-9. [http://dx.doi.org/10.1128/JVI.01650-06]

[67] Lazear HM, Pinto AK, Ramos HJ, *et al.* Pattern recognition receptor MDA5 modulates CD8+ T cell-dependent clearance of West Nile virus from the central nervous system. J Virol 2013; 87(21): 11401-15. [http://dx.doi.org/10.1128/JVI.01403-13]

[68] Shrestha B, Pinto AK, Green S, Bosch I, Diamond MS. CD8+ T cells use TRAIL to restrict West Nile virus pathogenesis by controlling infection in neurons. J Virol 2012; 86(17): 8937-48. [http://dx.doi.org/10.1128/JVI.00673-12]

[69] Shrestha B, Samuel MA, Diamond MS. CD8+ T cells require perforin to clear West Nile virus from infected neurons. J Virol 2006; 80(1): 119-29. [http://dx.doi.org/10.1128/JVI.80.1.119-129.2006]

[70] Shrestha B, Diamond MS. Fas ligand interactions contribute to CD8+ T-cell-mediated control of West Nile virus infection in the central nervous system. J Virol 2007; 81(21): 11749-57. [http://dx.doi.org/10.1128/JVI.01136-07]

[71] Samuel MA, Diamond MS. Alpha/beta interferon protects against lethal West Nile virus infection by restricting cellular tropism and enhancing neuronal survival. J Virol 2005; 79(21): 13350-61. [http://dx.doi.org/10.1128/JVI.79.21.13350-13361.2005]

[72] Shrestha B, Wang T, Samuel MA, *et al.* Gamma interferon plays a crucial early antiviral role in protection against West Nile virus infection. J Virol 2006; 80(11): 5338-48. [http://dx.doi.org/10.1128/JVI.00274-06]

[73] Town T, Bai F, Wang T, *et al.* Toll-like receptor 7 mitigates lethal West Nile encephalitis *via* interleukin 23-dependent immune cell infiltration and homing. Immunity 2009; 30(2): 242-53.

[http://dx.doi.org/10.1016/j.immuni.2008.11.012]

[74] Gubler DJ. The continuing spread of West Nile virus in the western hemisphere. Clin Infect Dis 2007; 45: 1039-46.

[75] Davis CT, Ebel GD, Lanciotti RS, Brault AC, Guzman H, Siirin M. Phylogenetic analysis of North American West Nile virus isolates, 2001–2004: evidence for the emergence of a dominant genotype. Virology 2005; 342: 252-65.

[76] Lanciotti RS, Roehrig JT, Deubel V, Smith J, Parker M, Steele K. Origin of the West Nile virus responsible for an outbreak of encephalitis in the northeastern United States. Science 1999; 286: 2333-7.

[77] Kelley TW, Prayson RA, Ruiz AI, Isada CM, Gordon SM. The neuropathology of West Nile virus meningoencephalitis. A report of two cases and review of the literature. Am J Clin Pathol 2003; 119: 749-53.

[78] Town T, Bai F, Wang T, Kaplan AT, Qian F, Montgomery RR. Toll-like receptor 7 mitigates lethal West Nile encephalitis *via* interleukin 23-dependent immune cell infiltration and homing. Immunity 2009; 30: 242-53.

[79] Wang T, Town T, Alexopoulou L, Anderson JF, Fikrig E, Flavell RA. Toll-like receptor 3 mediates West Nile virus entry into the brain causing lethal encephalitis. Nat Med 2004; 10: 1366-73.

[80] Fang H. Thomas Welte, Xin Zheng, Gwong-Jen J. Chang, Michael R. Holbrook, Lynn Soong, Tian Wang, γδd T cells promote the maturation of dendritic cells during West Nile virus infection. FEMS Immunol Med Microbiol 2010; 59(1): 71-80.
[http://dx.doi.org/10.1111/j.1574-695X.2010.00663.x]

[81] Chugh PE, Damania BA, Dittmer DP. Toll-like receptor-3 is dispensable for the innate microRNA response to West Nile virus (WNV). PLoS One 2014; 9(8)e104770
[http://dx.doi.org/10.1371/journal.pone.0104770]

[82] Fredericksen BL, Keller BC, Fornek J, Katze MG, Gale M Jr. Establishment and maintenance of the innate antiviral response to West Nile Virus involves both RIG-I and MDA5 signaling through IPS-1. J Virol 2008; 82(2): 609-16.
[http://dx.doi.org/10.1128/JVI.01305-07]

[83] Zhang HL, Ye HQ, Liu SQ, *et al.* West Nile Virus NS1 Antagonizes Interferon Beta Production by Targeting RIG-I and MDA5. J Virol 2017; 91(18): e02396-16.
[http://dx.doi.org/10.1128/JVI.02396-16]

[84] Town T, Bai F, Wang T, *et al.* Toll-like receptor 7 mitigates lethal West Nile encephalitis *via* interleukin 23-dependent immune cell infiltration and homing. Immunity 2009; 30(2): 242-53.
[http://dx.doi.org/10.1016/j.immuni.2008.11.012]

[85] Sabouri AH, Marcondes MC, Flynn C, *et al.* TLR signaling controls lethal encephalitis in WNV-infected brain. Brain Res 2014; 1574: 84-95.
[http://dx.doi.org/10.1016/j.brainres.2014.05.049]

CHAPTER 9

Japanese Encephalitis and Toll-like Receptors

Abstract: Viral encephalitis is a major pathological situation. It can be caused either by DNA or RNA viruses. Japanese encephalitis belongs to the member of *flavivirus* and it is a mosquito-borne disease, causing viral disease. Japanese encephalitis can be prevented by a vaccine. TLR3 and TLR4 signal pathways are activated due to JE Japanese encephalitis infection. TLR3 and Retinoic acid-inducible I also participate in mediating inflammation owing to Japanese encephalitis infection. In this kind of virus infection first, the cells are infected, causing primary viremia, subsequently infecting the CNS tissues as well. More than 60% of the world's population is living in JE endemic places.

Keywords: CNS inflammation, Flavirius infections, Murine microglia cells, TLR7 mRNA levels.

INTRODUCTION

Due to climate change and global warming, this disease is now spreading to various parts of the world where previously it was not reported [1]. Approximately 60% of the population is living in endemic countries. There are four genera of *flaviviruses* that are very lethal to human beings, namely, *Pegvirus*, *Pestivirus*, *Flavivirus*, and *Hepacivirus*. Viruses such as dengue virus (DENV), West Nile virus (WNV), Zika virus (ZIKV), and Japanese encephalitis virus (JEV) are pathogenic to humans and fall in *flaviviruses*. As per WHO, approximately 67,000 cases occur in JE endemic countries every year despite vaccination progress [2]. JE can cause mortality in 30% of cases, and survivors of this disease face cognitive impairment, and motor paralysis as a result of neurological squeal [3].

TLRs in Japanese encephalitis (JE) have not been well explored. There was a study in which TLR knockout mice displayed differential immune responses [4]. It was found that TLR3 -/- was highly susceptible to JE infection whereas TLR4-/ - mice displayed resistance.In most cases of flavirius infections, TLR 7 plays the first line of defence by recognising the pathogen. In systemic infection, TLR7 activation produces Type I interferon production, which in turn protects the mice from the JE virus by creating an antiviral state [4]. Post-JEV infection, TLR7

Jayalakshmi Krishnan

mRNA levels were elevated,this further was confirmed by TLR-/- mice, wherein TLR7-/- mice displayed a very high viral load [5]. TLR8 was found to be highly regulated in TLR7-/- knockout mice, which may act as a parallel immune protecting effect to JE infection in the absence of TLR7. TLR polymorphism plays an important role in the susceptibility of JE patients to the virus. For example, Leu412Phe polymorphism, with high frequency was noted in JE patients in contrast to the control group [6].

Type I interferon production creates an antiviral state in the JEV-infected cells through TLR7 thus offering a protective effect [7]. Several studies on TLR-/- were done in mice to understand the effects of JEV. Mice with TLR 3 KO condition display high susceptibility whereas mice with TLR 4 KO condition have shown high resistance to JE. These differences primarily lie in eliciting pathological reactions. Severe CNS inflammation and infiltration of monocytes ($CD11b^{+}Ly\text{-}6C^{high}$) were attributed to the increased viral burden in the TLR3 KO condition. In addition, there was increased Blood Brain Barrier permeability leading to cytokine and chemokine expression in various cells [4]. On the other hand, TLR4 KO mice display less CNS inflammation by reduced pro-inflammatory cytokine expression characterised by less viral burden and little leukocyte infiltration. Although JE can be curable by Vaccination, still much research needs to be done on its interaction with the immune system. Toll-like receptors 7 and 8 play an important role in sensing the viral components of JEV thus priming the immune cells [8]. In brain cells such as microglial cells TLRs 3, 2 and 7 interact with the JE virus [9].

In murine microglia cells, KO of TLR3 and infection with JEV lead to high viral load [10]. TLR3 and retinoic acid-inducible gene I (RIG-I) in microglia cells play an important role in JEV pathogenesis. These two molecules can recognise ds RNA which in turn leads to the upregulation of extracellular signal-regulated kinase (ERK) and p38 mitogen-activated protein kinase (p38MAPK) along with TLR3 expression. These molecules were abrogated along with activator protein 1 (AP-1), and nuclear factor κB (NF-κB) when TLR3 and RIG-I were attenuated. The effects of TLR 3 and RIG 1 KO is: Increased viral proliferation and reduction of TNF-α, IL-6, and CCL-2 secretion usually induced by JEV [10].

Endosomal compartments have TLR7 and TLR8, these receptors sense the ssRNA viruses. Along with TLRs, RNA helicases also take part in sensing the viral accumulation in the cytosol. For example, RIG-I (retonic acid inducible gene -1) recognises all RNA viruses such as paramyxoviruses, influenza virus, and Japanese encephalitis virus and other viruses such as paramyxoviruses and influenza virus [11, 12]. JEV also stops the cross-presentation of both soluble and cell-associated antigens by activating the TLR2-MyD88 and p38 MAPK-signalling [13, 14]. This suppression of cross-presentation can lead to diminished $CD8^+$ T-cell responses to antigens. In order to plan an effective vaccine strategy, understanding these TLR-mediated responses would be better.

JEV and Inflammation Through TLRs

During systemic infection, using knock-down mice (TLR7(KD), it was demonstrated that JEV infections lead to the production of type I IFN production leading to protection by establishing an antiviral state.The role of microRNAs has been also identified in causing microglial activation in the Japanese Encephalitis virus (JEV) infection. In JEV-infected microglial cells, let-7a and let-7b (let-7a/b) have been overexpressed leading to the caspase activation and cell death which was mediated by the NOTCH-TLR7 pathway [15]. In human microglial cells also the same kind of observation was made that the JE virus uses microRNAs to achieve cell death [16]. In a study, JEV-infected neuro2a cell line and adult mice were used to understand the patterns of innate immune mechanisms. In TLR3 gene silencing conditions in both cell lines and mice, there was a higher replication of JEV irus with MyD88 and IRF 7 overexpression [17]. CNS of JEV-infected mice upon microarray studies showed higher expression of TLR2, TLR4, and TLR7. In humans, upon mild and severe infection with JEV, it was found that significant upregulation of chemokine and TLR7 was observed that may be considered as significant tools for viral inflammation [18]. Compensatory roles for TLRs knockout were also identified in mice. It was found that in TLR7-/- mice, there was a significant upregulation of TLR8, indicating that there is a compensatory role created by the TLR7 knockout condition. Among mild and severely infected JE patients it was shown that differential expression of Chemokine ligands and TLRs are noted as higher. Using the infected dendrite cells and macrophages the JE virus enters the brain through newly produced virion particles. Culex mosquitoes spread the JE infection from bird to bird and also to other animals and humans in tropical countries [19]. In the temperate regions vertical transmission of JEV is also higher [20, 21]. In $CD8^+$ T cells, TLR2-MyD88 and p38 MAPK signal pathway mediate the cross-presentation of soluble antigens from the JE virus [22]. Dendritic cells were impaired due to JE infection with very poor CD 4 and CD8 cell responses. These effects are mediated by both MyD88-dependent and independent pathways leading to viral survival. In macrophages JE induced chemokine and proinflammatory cytokines mRNA.

MicroRNAs and JEV

There was an involvement of microRNAs in JEV infection to regulate the inflammation creased by JEV virus. The *in vitro* and *in vivo* studies on miRNA show that miR-19b-3p has been elevated in the cultured cells and in mice brain after the infection with the JE virus. This elevated miRNAs were involved in producing higher inflammatory status of the cells by up regulating inflammatory mediators such as TNFa, Interleukins and chemokines. However, silencing of miR-19b-3p has completely abrogated the inflammatory responses. This inflammatory mechanism of miRNA is mediated through the ring finger protein 11 which is am negative regulator of the NFKB protein [23].

Src-family tyrosine kinases especially Ras/Raf/extracellular signal-regulated kinase (ERK), have also been reported to be active mediator of the infection and inflammation mediated through the JEV. The microglial cells infected with JEV have shown higher levels of inflammatory mediators such as TNF a, interleukins and chemokines by activating NF-kB [24]. RANTES (regulated upon activation, normal T cell expressed and secreted) levels were higher in astrocytes and microglial cells exposed to JE virus. In addition, cells stimulated with TNF and interleukins express high levels of RANTES gene expression and other factors such as ROS and ERKs [25].JEV infection modulated the tyrosine kinases activity by phosphorylating the Src protein tyrosine kinase (PTK) function in neuronal and glail cell cultures [26]. Similar studies of higher levels of inflammatory mediators are seen in microglail cells infected with JEV. The microglia activation is evidenced by higher levels of RANTES production, Interleukins such s IL1 and IL6 followed by TNF alpha levels [27]. PTK inhibitor studies in neurons and glial cells have shown that these inhibitors were able to reduce the TNF alpha levels and interleukin levels. Treatment of microglial and neuronal cells with PTK inhibitors such as enistein, herbimycin A, and PP2 have not stopped JEV replication but have caused the cells to cease the neurotoxicity caused by JE virus [28].

Microglial Cells /MicroRNA and JEV

Involvement of microglial cells in the inflammation mediated by JEV was studied in BV2 cells. The microaary experiments were done for 6, 12, and 24 h after the infection of JEV in BV.2 cells. There was a production of 212 proteins out of which MyD88 was not shown to be elevated even IRAK1, IRAK4, and TRAF6 were not up regulated. But surprising TLR2 mediated signal transduction pathways such as TLR2, PI3K, and AKT were elevated proving the JEV can cause the activation of TLR2 and lead to the inflammatory mechanisms [29]. microRNAs such as miR-155 and miR-146a were involved in the inflammation mediated by JEV virus in microglia CHME3 cells by expressing high levels of complement factor H (CFH) and interferon regulatory factor 8 (IRF8). miR-155 over expressing cells display elvelaated CD 45 and Activators of Transcription (p-STAT1) expression [30]. JEV activates the Matrix metalloproteinases in rat brain. In RBA-1 cells the JEV has induced the expression of MMP9 to lead to

NFKB activation and production of ROS and p38 MAPK, JNK1/2,and p42/p44 MAPK [31]. microRNAs such as miR-15b is elevated in mouse brain and glail cells upon infection with JEV. Ring finger protein 125 (RNF125) seems to be the target for the miR-15b mediated inflammatory changes in JEV infection [32]. miR-146a levels were elevated in BALB/c mice brain upon JEV infection with the increasing levels of various proinflammatory cytokines [33]. Microglial cells were exposed to two different kinds of strains of JEV . Theyy are 1) JaOArS982 and 2) P20778. The studies show that miR-146a levels were elevated. At the same time there was a decrease in the production of IRAK1, IRAK2, TRAF6, and STAT1 genes. miR-155 was seen to be highly expressed during JEV infection in BV2 glail cells [34]. miR-301a targets NF-κB-repressing factor (NKRF) to augment the inflammation caused by JEV in microglail cells [35].

CONCLUDING REMARKS

Before infecting the CNS, JEV multiplies in macrophages and other antigen-presenting cells such as dendritic cells (DCs) (Kurane 2002). Upon infection by JE the $CD8\alpha^{+}CD11c^{+}$ DCs cells, display modulation in their functions through the MyD88 adaptor molecule of TLRs [13]. Through a study on $CD8\alpha^{+}CD11c^{+}$ DCs that lacked TLR2, TLR3, TLR9, and MyD88 molecules in different strains of mice suppressed cross-presentation of soluble OVA protein was seen in TLR3 and TLR9 KO mice. On the other hand, both TLR2 and MyD88 KO did not show any impaired cross-presentation this indicates that MyD88 is involved in the inhibition of cross-presentation.

CONSENT FOR PUBLICATION

Not applicable.

CONFLICT OF INTEREST

The author declares no conflict of interest, financial or otherwise.

ACKNOWLEDGEMENT

Declared none.

REFERENCES

[1] Mackenzie JS, Gubler DJ, Petersen LR. Emerging *flaviviruses*: the spread and resurgence of Japanese encephalitis, West Nile and dengue viruses. Nat Med 2004; 10(S12) (Suppl.): S98-S109. [http://dx.doi.org/10.1038/nm1144] [PMID: 15577938]

[2] Luvira V, Chamnanchanunt S, Thanachartwet V, Phumratanaprapin W, Viriyavejakul A. Cerebral venous sinus thrombosis in severe malaria. Southeast Asian J Trop Med Public Health 2009; 40(5): 893-7. [PMID: 19842369].
[PMID: 19842369]

[3] Temperley ND, Berlin S, Paton IR, Griffin DK, Burt DW. Evolution of the chicken Toll-like receptor gene family: A story of gene gain and gene loss. BMC Genomics 2008; 9(1): 62. [http://dx.doi.org/10.1186/1471-2164-9-62] [PMID: 18241342]

[4] Han YW, Choi JY, Uyangaa E, *et al.* Distinct dictation of Japanese encephalitis virus-induced neuroinflammation and lethality *via* triggering TLR3 and TLR4 signal pathways. PLoS Pathog 2014; 10(9)e1004319 [http://dx.doi.org/10.1371/journal.ppat.1004319] [PMID: 25188232]

[5] Awais M, Wang K, Lin X, *et al.* TLR7 deficiency leads to TLR8 compensative regulation of immune response against JEV in mice. Front Immunol 2017; 8(FEB): 160. [http://dx.doi.org/10.3389/fimmu.2017.00160] [PMID: 28265274]

[6] Biyani S, Garg RK, Jain A, *et al.* Toll-like receptor-3 gene polymorphism in patients with Japanese encephalitis. J Neuroimmunol 2015; 286(8): 71-6. [http://dx.doi.org/10.1016/j.jneuroim.2015.07.010] [PMID: 26298326]

[7] Nazmi A, Mukherjee S, Kundu K, *et al.* TLR7 is a key regulator of innate immunity against Japanese encephalitis virus infection. Neurobiol Dis 2014; 69(1): 235-47. [http://dx.doi.org/10.1016/j.nbd.2014.05.036] [PMID: 24909816]

[8] Lannes N, Summerfield A, Filgueira L. Regulation of inflammation in Japanese encephalitis. J Neuroinflammation 2017; 14(1): 158. [http://dx.doi.org/10.1186/s12974-017-0931-5] [PMID: 28807053]

[9] Fadnis PR, Ravi V, Desai A, Turtle L, Solomon T. Innate immune mechanisms in Japanese encephalitis virus infection: effect on transcription of pattern recognition receptors in mouse neuronal cells and brain tissue. Viral Immunol 2013; 26(6): 366-77. [http://dx.doi.org/10.1089/vim.2013.0016] [PMID: 24236856]

[10] Jiang R, Ye J, Zhu B, Song Y, Chen H, Cao S. Roles of TLR3 and RIG-I in mediating the inflammatory response in mouse microglia following Japanese encephalitis virus infection. J Immunol Res 2014; 2014(1): 1-11. [http://dx.doi.org/10.1155/2014/787023] [PMID: 25101306]

[11] Mizuno Y, Kato Y, Kanagawa S, *et al.* A case of postmalaria neurological syndrome in Japan. J Infect Chemother 2006; 12(6): 399-401. [http://dx.doi.org/10.1016/S1341-321X(06)70902-3] [PMID: 17235648]

[12] Kato H, Takeuchi O, Sato S, *et al.* Differential roles of MDA5 and RIG-I helicases in the recognition of RNA viruses. Nature 2006; 441(7089): 101-5. [http://dx.doi.org/10.1038/nature04734] [PMID: 16625202]

[13] Aleyas AG, George JA, Han YW, *et al.* Functional modulation of dendritic cells and macrophages by Japanese encephalitis virus through MyD88 adaptor molecule-dependent and -independent pathways. J Immunol 2009; 183(4): 2462-74. [http://dx.doi.org/10.4049/jimmunol.0801952] [PMID: 19635909]

[14] Aleyas AG, Han YW, Patil AM, Kim SB, Kim K, Eo SK. Impaired cross-presentation of CD8α $^{+}$ CD11c $^{+}$ dendritic cells by Japanese encephalitis virus in a TLR2/MyD88 signal pathway-dependent manner. Eur J Immunol 2012; 42(10): 2655-66. [http://dx.doi.org/10.1002/eji.201142052] [PMID: 22706912]

[15] Mukherjee S, Akbar I, Kumari B, Vrati S, Basu A, Banerjee A. Japanese Encephalitis Virus-induced *let-7a/b* interacted with the NOTCH-TLR 7 pathway in microglia and facilitated neuronal death *via* caspase activation. J Neurochem 2019; 149(4): 518-34. [http://dx.doi.org/10.1111/jnc.14645] [PMID: 30556910]

[16] Rastogi M, Srivastava N, Singh SK. Exploitation of microRNAs by Japanese Encephalitis virus in human microglial cells. J Med Virol 2018; 90(4): 648-54. [http://dx.doi.org/10.1002/jmv.24995] [PMID: 29149532]

[17] Gupta N, Rao PVL. Transcriptomic profile of host response in Japanese encephalitis virus infection. Virol J 2011; 8(1): 92.
[http://dx.doi.org/10.1186/1743-422X-8-92] [PMID: 21371334]

[18] Chowdhury P, Khan SA. Differential Expression Levels of Inflammatory Chemokines and *TLR* s in Patients Suffering from Mild and Severe Japanese Encephalitis. Viral Immunol 2019; 32(1): 68-74.
[http://dx.doi.org/10.1089/vim.2018.0103] [PMID: 30585774]

[19] Samy AM, Alkishe AA, Thomas SM, Wang L, Zhang W. Mapping the potential distributions of etiological agent, vectors, and reservoirs of Japanese Encephalitis in Asia and Australia. Acta Trop 2018; 188: 108-17.
[http://dx.doi.org/10.1016/j.actatropica.2018.08.014] [PMID: 30118701]

[20] Pearce JC, Learoyd TP, Langendorf BJ, Logan JG. Japanese encephalitis: the vectors, ecology and potential for expansion. J Travel Med 2018; 25 (Suppl. 1): S16-26.
[http://dx.doi.org/10.1093/jtm/tay009] [PMID: 29718435]

[21] Zhao S, Lou Y, Chiu APY, He D. Modelling the skip-and-resurgence of Japanese encephalitis epidemics in Hong Kong. J Theor Biol 2018; 454: 1-10.
[http://dx.doi.org/10.1016/j.jtbi.2018.05.017] [PMID: 29792875]

[22] Aleyas AG, Han YW, Patil AM, Kim SB, Kim K, Eo SK. Impaired cross-presentation of CD8α $^+$ CD11c $^+$ dendritic cells by Japanese encephalitis virus in a TLR2/MyD88 signal pathway-dependent manner. Eur J Immunol 2012; 42(10): 2655-66.
[http://dx.doi.org/10.1002/eji.201142052] [PMID: 22706912]

[23] Ashraf U, Zhu B, Ye J, *et al.* MicroRNA-19b-3p Modulates Japanese Encephalitis Virus-Mediated Inflammation *via* Targeting RNF11. J Virol 2016; 90(9): 4780-95.
[http://dx.doi.org/10.1128/JVI.02586-15] [PMID: 26937036]

[24] Chen CJ, Ou YC, Chang CY, *et al.* Src signaling involvement in Japanese encephalitis virus-induced cytokine production in microglia. Neurochem Int 2011; 58(8): 924-33.
[http://dx.doi.org/10.1016/j.neuint.2011.02.022] [PMID: 21354239]

[25] Chen CJ, Ou YC, Chang CY, *et al.* TNF-α and IL-1β mediate Japanese encephalitis virus-induced RANTES gene expression in astrocytes. Neurochem Int 2011; 58(2): 234-42.
[http://dx.doi.org/10.1016/j.neuint.2010.12.009] [PMID: 21167894]

[26] Raung SL, Chen SY, Liao SL, Chen JH, Chen CJ. Japanese encephalitis virus infection stimulates Src tyrosine kinase in neuron/glia. Neurosci Lett 2007; 419(3): 263-8.
[http://dx.doi.org/10.1016/j.neulet.2007.04.036] [PMID: 17493752]

[27] Chen CJ, Ou YC, Lin SY, *et al.* Glial activation involvement in neuronal death by Japanese encephalitis virus infection. J Gen Virol 2010; 91(4): 1028-37.
[http://dx.doi.org/10.1099/vir.0.013565-0] [PMID: 20007359]

[28] Raung SL, Chen SY, Liao SL, Chen JH, Chen CJ. Tyrosine kinase inhibitors attenuate Japanese encephalitis virus-induced neurotoxicity. Biochem Biophys Res Commun 2005; 327(2): 399-406.
[http://dx.doi.org/10.1016/j.bbrc.2004.12.034] [PMID: 15629129]

[29] Zhao G, Gao Y, Zhang J, *et al.* Toll-like receptor 2 signaling pathway activation contributes to a highly efficient inflammatory response in Japanese encephalitis virus-infected mouse microglial cells by proteomics. Front Microbiol 2022; 13989183
[http://dx.doi.org/10.3389/fmicb.2022.989183] [PMID: 36171749]

[30] Pareek S, Roy S, Kumari B, Jain P, Banerjee A, Vrati S. miR-155 induction in microglial cells suppresses Japanese encephalitis virus replication and negatively modulates innate immune responses. J Neuroinflammation 2014; 11(1): 97.
[http://dx.doi.org/10.1186/1742-2094-11-97] [PMID: 24885259]

[31] Tung WH, Tsai HW, Lee IT, *et al.* Japanese encephalitis virus induces matrix metalloproteinase-9 in rat brain astrocytes *via* NF-κB signalling dependent on MAPKs and reactive oxygen species. Br J

Pharmacol 2010; 161(7): 1566-83.
[http://dx.doi.org/10.1111/j.1476-5381.2010.00982.x] [PMID: 20698853]

[32] Zhu B, Ye J, Nie Y, *et al.* MicroRNA-15b Modulates Japanese Encephalitis Virus–Mediated Inflammation *via* Targeting RNF125. J Immunol 2015; 195(5): 2251-62.
[http://dx.doi.org/10.4049/jimmunol.1500370] [PMID: 26202983]

[33] Deng M, Du G, Zhao J, Du X. miR-146a negatively regulates the induction of proinflammatory cytokines in response to Japanese encephalitis virus infection in microglial cells. Arch Virol 2017; 162(6): 1495-505.
[http://dx.doi.org/10.1007/s00705-017-3226-3] [PMID: 28190197]

[34] Thounaojam MC, Kundu K, Kaushik DK, *et al.* MicroRNA 155 regulates Japanese encephalitis virus-induced inflammatory response by targeting Src homology 2-containing inositol phosphatase 1. J Virol 2014; 88(9): 4798-810.
[http://dx.doi.org/10.1128/JVI.02979-13] [PMID: 24522920]

[35] Hazra B, Chakraborty S, Bhaskar M, Mukherjee S, Mahadevan A, Basu A. miR-301a Regulates Inflammatory Response to Japanese Encephalitis Virus Infection *via* Suppression of NKRF Activity. J Immunol 2019; 203(8): 2222-38.
[http://dx.doi.org/10.4049/jimmunol.1900003] [PMID: 31527198]

SUBJECT INDEX

Jayalakshmi Krishnan

C

D

E

F

G

H

K

L

M

V

W

Y

www.ingramcontent.com/pod-product-compliance
Lightning Source LLC
LaVergne TN
LVHW070137110826
845147LV00002B/269